D1238642

ADVANCE PRAISE FOR *THE VOID INSIDE*

"Professor Pamela Keel is the world's foremost expert on purging disorder. In *The Void Inside*, she provides a riveting account of two decades of scientific discovery that have shaped our understanding of an eating disorder that affects millions. This book is an absolute must-read for professionals, patients, and carers."

—**Jennifer J. Thomas**, PhD, Co-Director, Eating Disorders
Clinical and Research Program, Massachusetts
General Hospital, Harvard Medical School

"This book, written by the world's leading authority, provides a comprehensive summary of Purging Disorder. It combines a thorough discussion of the its characteristics with detailed descriptions of individuals who have struggled with it. This definitive volume on Purging Disorder is a critical and welcome resource for patients, practitioners, and researchers."

—**B. Timothy Walsh**, MD, Professor of Psychiatry,
Columbia University

The Void Inside

Bringing Purging Disorder to Light

PAMELA K. KEEL

OXFORD
UNIVERSITY PRESS

Oxford University Press is a department of the University of Oxford. It furthers
the University's objective of excellence in research, scholarship, and education
by publishing worldwide. Oxford is a registered trade mark of Oxford University
Press in the UK and certain other countries.

Published in the United States of America by Oxford University Press
198 Madison Avenue, New York, NY 10016, United States of America.

© Oxford University Press 2020

Library of Congress Cataloging-in-Publication Data
Names: Keel, Pamela K., 1970– author.
Title: The void inside : bringing purging disorder to light / Pamela K. Keel.
Description: New York, NY : Oxford University Press, [2020] |
Includes bibliographical references and index.
Identifiers: LCCN 2020008764 (print) | LCCN 2020008765 (ebook) |
ISBN 9780190061166 (hardback) | ISBN 9780190061180 (epub) |
ISBN 9780190061197
Subjects: LCSH: Eating disorders. | Vomiting.
Classification: LCC RC552.E18 K445 2020 (print) | LCC RC552.E18 (ebook) |
DDC 616.85/26—dc23
LC record available at https://lccn.loc.gov/2020008764
LC ebook record available at https://lccn.loc.gov/2020008765

9 8 7 6 5 4 3 2 1
Printed by Sheridan Books, Inc., United States of America

CONTENTS

ACKNOWLEDGMENTS

A book with a single author reflects the efforts of a lot of people. I want to start by thanking my editor, Sarah Harrington, who has provided guidance, support, critical feedback, and enthusiasm at the exact times needed, as well as the staff at Oxford University Press, including Hayley Singer and Wendy Walker, for their work in bringing this book together. A special thanks to Anne Becker, M.D., Ph.D., who shared her contact in Fiji so that I could learn more about purging in this culture. I also want to thank every researcher who answered my calls to study purging disorder. Their efforts have significantly advanced knowledge on this problem, and I hope this book inspires future work to understand and eliminate this illness. Finally, I want to thank every person with purging disorder who has sought treatment, volunteered for research, and shared their experiences with me by phone or e-mail. I have learned so much from you.

I have had what you refer to as purging disorder for 8 years. Generally I don't actually view it as a problem but I am able to recognize that vomiting 10 times a day is not normal behaviour [. . .] I have been to therapists, psychiatrists, group therapy in [. . .] none of which have been effective. [. . .] I know I have done some serious damage to my body and sometimes I feel that I'm completely losing my mind. [. . .] I don't want to die and I'm pretty sure blood in the vomit isn't a good thing.

E-mail received September 2007

This message reveals several truths about purging disorder: the severe and enduring nature of the illness, the emotional and physical toll of purging, and the fear that purging will cause death. There is uncertainty as to whether purging, even ten times a day for eight years, is a problem, and the pressing need for treatment that works. What the e-mail doesn't reveal is that most people with purging disorder never seek treatment. Many ask, "If I don't have anorexia or bulimia, do I have a 'real' disorder?" They do. But their disorder has remained hidden.

Purging disorder existed long before I first encountered it, but it went unrecognized—unrecognized by the field of mental health, by those with the disorder, and by everyone around them. Individuals with purging disorder do not look different on the outside, and the purging is done in secret. Yet, the ease with which purging disorder eludes detection should not be taken as evidence that it is rare or insignificant. Right now, more than 2 million girls and women suffer from purging disorder in the United States, and nearly half a million boys and men join them. These numbers grow exponentially when we count cases of purging disorder worldwide. But any accounting of those currently affected underestimates the disorder's full impact because it does not include those who have died. A recent study found 11 deaths in nine years among 219 purging disorder patients. One or two individuals might have been expected to die over this period, making 11 deaths shocking.

When I began my work on purging disorder in 1998, it was not even a named condition. How did I get interested in an eating disorder without a definition or even a name? Three events propelled me—all during my first year as an assistant professor at Harvard University. I was 28 years old and writing articles based on my doctoral dissertation—a long-term follow-up study of bulimia. For women who remained ill, I wanted to know if they still had bulimia or if their disorder had evolved into something else, such as binge-eating disorder—a newly proposed syndrome appearing in the fourth edition of the *Diagnostic and Statistical Manual of Mental Disorders*[1] (DSM-IV). Women diagnosed with bulimia 10 to 15 years before were 10 times more likely to still have bulimia than to cross over to either anorexia or binge-eating disorder. This supported the notion that bulimia wasn't just a phase of another eating disorder. However, I also found that these individuals were now just as likely to purge without bingeing as they were to binge and purge. Purging without bingeing meant they no longer met full criteria for bulimia, but they didn't seem to have meaningfully recovered. If they weren't recovered, did they still have bulimia or had they developed a different eating disorder?

During that same year, I started a clinical fellowship in psychiatry at Massachusetts General Hospital. Every Friday, I took the Red Line from Porter Square to Mass General, where I completed a weekly intake assessment and followed a small caseload of patients in the Eating Disorders Program. The first three women I met were within a healthy weight range, ruling out a diagnosis of anorexia. None reported binge-eating episodes, ruling out a diagnosis of bulimia or binge-eating disorder. But all three induced vomiting after eating normal amounts of food and expressed an intense fear of gaining weight. I began treating one of these women,[2] Cara (name changed), a 27-year-old secretary who described vomiting when she ate more than a single packet of plain oatmeal with a cup of nonfat plain yogurt. For example, when Cara went out for brunch with friends, she would have to excuse herself partway through the meal so she could vomit everything she had eaten. What treatment should I offer? Should I treat her as if she had anorexia, a disorder for which treatment focuses on weight restoration, even though her weight was fine and there were no clear evidence-based treatments for adults? Or should I treat her as if she had bulimia, a disorder for which the first line of treatment was cognitive-behavioral therapy (CBT)? Given these options, I chose CBT, but it didn't fit. Working through the treatment, I kept running into a wall because of CBT's focus on stopping the binge eating, a symptom Cara did not have. For example, CBT for bulimia emphasized that " 'binges' usually involve the consumption of a large number of calories (it can be salutary for patients to calculate the calorie content of a typical binge) and that self-induced vomiting does not retrieve everything that has been eaten."[3] Further, "vomiting *per se* does not need to be tackled, since in the great majority of cases it ceases once the patient has stopped overeating."[4] I found the world's best resource on bulimia treatment to be astoundingly unhelpful. Why? Because my patient didn't have bulimia. But I wouldn't understand that until a few years later.

The third fateful experience occurred while recruiting participants for a study I designed to learn more about binge-eating disorder. My undergraduate research assistants plastered Cambridge with posters asking, "Do you binge?"[5] We received a robust response but noticed that the *size* of binge episodes rendered many callers ineligible. One in five callers described a loss of control while eating amounts of food that were not larger than what others would eat. For example, one women reported a loss of control after eating a blueberry muffin for breakfast. More alarming, over 70% were compensating for these "binges" by purging. Few things are more frustrating than turning away prospective study participants because they don't have the right disorder. Instead, they had an eating disorder that no one had yet studied because their behaviors did not fit neatly within the boundaries of our diagnostic definitions.

I can't say how my career would have turned out differently if all three of these experiences had not occurred during that first year. I only know what did happen.

By June 1, 1999, I submitted a grant application to the National Institute of Mental Health. The scope was modest. I wasn't aiming to identify a new disorder. Instead, I was convinced the problem was that bulimia's definition was too narrow. Did we really think that a woman who felt compelled to vomit after eating three cookies had a less severe eating disorder than a woman who vomited after eating an entire package of cookies? I received a small project grant to determine whether size mattered in defining binge episodes among normal-weight women who purged. In 2001, I published a paper on what I then called "subjective bulimia nervosa." I used the adjective "subjective" because the women *subjectively* felt that they had eaten too much before purging even though *objectively* they had not consumed more than most healthy people would eat.[6] Key findings supported that "subjective bulimia nervosa" was just as pathological as bulimia but that those with bulimia had greater impulsiveness around food and across multiple areas of their lives. These findings shifted my thinking and the terms and labels I used. From 2001 to 2005, I shifted away from using "subjective bulimia nervosa" when I presented at conferences. My data indicated it was more than a simple variant of bulimia. Although the amount of food women ate before purging was not critical for establishing a clinically significant disorder, it might represent a meaningful boundary between disorders. This boundary might reflect differences in personality traits and biology that would reveal the underlying causes of both disorders.

This new disorder required a name, and I called it "purging disorder" in all subsequent publications. Reports of purging disorder started appearing from around the world, as the field recognized the alarmingly high numbers of people who purged without bingeing and who were not underweight. In 2013, the American Psychiatric Association published the fifth edition of the DSM (DSM-5), and a newly named condition appears on page 353: purging disorder. It is uniquely characterized by "recurrent purging to influence weight or shape (e.g., self-induced vomiting; misuse of laxatives, diuretics, or other medications) in the absence of binge eating."[7]

Recently my former student K. Jean Forney, Ph.D., completed a long-term follow-up study of purging disorder for her doctoral dissertation. In addition to describing how women were doing 10 years following first diagnosis, she compared outcomes to bulimia. My patient Cara is one of the participants in this study, and I am pleased to share that she is doing well. However, she is in the minority. More than a decade after initial diagnosis, over 60% of individuals with purging disorder still struggle with their illness. Cara was also an exception because most never sought treatment for their eating disorder. As a group, they were significantly less likely to have ever received treatment compared to women with bulimia. The finding echoes results from my first article and reflects how a diagnosis (or the lack thereof) impacts treatment. This makes purging disorder's inclusion in the DSM-5 an important step forward. But it's not enough.

Purging disorder did not come into existence when I first encountered it. It had existed for decades, maybe centuries, and it had gone unrecognized for all of that time. In her memoir, *Purge: Rehab Diaries*, Nicole Johns wrote, "At 137 pounds, in the midst of consuming diet-pill cocktails, starving, and purging, I was hospitalized for fainting, a concussion, electrolyte imbalances, and three different kinds of heart-rhythm irregularities [. . .] but for a long time I refused to believe I had a problem because I was not underweight."[8] Compounding this, she was told by therapists, "I don't have an eating disorder" and "I'm not thin enough for treatment."[9] Individuals with purging disorder do not look different on the outside, and they neither eat too much (as in bulimia and binge-eating disorder) nor too little (as in anorexia)—so their eating behavior seems normal to most of us. The purging is done in secret, making it the easiest eating disorder to hide from others. You may think that you don't know anyone with purging disorder, but ask yourself how many people you have met over the course of your life. How many girls were in school with you? Based on national statistics for the United States, you probably were in middle school with over 300 girls and at high school with over 400 girls. Did you go to college? Add 15,000 women who shared a campus with you. How many had or went on to develop purging disorder? The alarming truth is that, statistically, it's almost certain that you have known someone with purging disorder.

Looking back, I recall times I probably encountered someone with purging disorder but failed to recognize it. My freshman year of college, a classmate shared that she had dreamed of being chased in circles by a fox and then vomiting gallons and gallons of vanilla ice cream. I asked her why she thought she had that dream. She answered, "Because I make myself vomit sometimes. It doesn't help me lose weight but it helps keep the weight off." So many things clicked into place—like the way she would get up while we were studying, grab her toothbrush and toothpaste, and head to the bathroom at the end of the hall. I just thought she was committed to oral hygiene, but she was actually vomiting nearly every evening we studied together. I didn't ask her anything more about it, and she didn't volunteer. Maybe she had bulimia or maybe she had purging disorder—again, I never probed for more information and wouldn't have known what to do with it if I had.

Even while collecting data for my dissertation I met women with purging disorder, but I didn't know what to do. As part of that long-term follow-up study of bulimia, I interviewed women and asked them to describe their symptoms from 10 to 15 years ago to confirm their diagnosis. Some of my participants described vomiting after ingesting normal amounts of food; they *never* had large binges, and they were never underweight. In the article published from this study, I wrote, "Of the 177 participants, 4 had never met full *DSM-IV* criteria for bulimia nervosa based on initial assessments and follow-up structured clinical interviews for

DSM-IV (SCID-I) and were eliminated from analyses, resulting in a sample size of 173 subjects."[10] Given the aims of that project, the decision made sense, but it reflects how I *eliminated* their data because they didn't fit into what I expected.

I received the following message after several major news outlets ran an Associated Press article on my research:

> I just read an article about research you have conducted/are doing regarding purging disorder. When I read the article it was the most amazing thing I've ever read because that is exactly what my problem is. I'm not bulimic or anorexic but I have the need to get rid of any normal amount of food I eat for many different reasons. I've never been able to explain to anyone exactly what it is that I feel I have. I've been through countless therapists etc and have never felt they truly understood my problem.
>
> *E-MAIL RECEIVED SEPTEMBER 2007*

Purging disorder has consumed the lives of too many for too long because it has operated in the periphery of awareness. The field has made great strides over the past 20 years in producing a wealth of data on purging disorder through both my own work and that of others. Although funding agencies require our findings to be publicly accessible, online access to an article written for fellow researchers doesn't make key information accessible to the public. It is imperative to translate this literature into an accessible and authoritative resource for those who suffer with the illness, their friends and loved ones, educators, health care professionals, and the general public. I wrote this book on purging disorder to help those affected with this illness by increasing awareness of what purging disorder is, what factors contribute to its unique development and maintenance, the outcomes associated with it, and what treatments work. This book is intended to bridge the gap between an urgent problem afflicting too many people and what we know about that problem.

A note about the title, *The Void Inside*—I chose this title to reflect both purging disorder's position within our health care system and its impact on individual people. Purging disorder inhabits the *void inside our diagnostic system*, occupying a space between anorexia and bulimia—being similar to each but not quite either. Purging disorder also creates a physical and emotional *void inside the individual* through the repeated act of purging unwanted calories and feelings. Bringing purging disorder to light is the first step toward replenishing what the illness has taken.

PART I

Emergence of a "New" Eating Disorder

Do We Need Another Eating Disorder?

When people learn I study eating disorders, they often ask about anorexia because this is the first eating disorder that comes to mind. For many, it's the *only* eating disorder that comes to mind. Out of curiosity, I searched Google for images of people with eating disorders. The first screen filled with 39 unique pictures (Figure 1.1). Of these, 95% of the people were young, 95% were white, 92% were female, 62% were underweight, and 3% were overweight (that is, one woman). The term "eating disorder" conjures up a powerful image of a young, emaciated white girl. This image has masked the different ways that eating can be disordered and who can be affected. If the Google search reflected reality, only 5% of the images would have been underweight, and they would have been far more diverse in terms of age, gender, race and ethnicity—but I'll get into that in the next chapter.

While all eating disorders involve a disturbance in eating, there are different ways that eating can be disturbed. These differences translate into meaningful distinctions in the central features of the disorders, when and where they emerge, how they impact the lives of those afflicted, and how they respond to treatment. Distinguishing among eating disorders is critical to understanding their causes and ultimately finding their cures. But if only 5% of eating disorders look like anorexia, what do the other ones look like and how many are there?

THE OFFICIAL EATING DISORDERS

There are three official eating disorders in the most recent edition of the American Psychiatric Association's *Diagnostic and Statistical Manual of Mental Disorders* (DSM-5).[1] These disorders include anorexia nervosa, bulimia nervosa, and binge-eating disorder (BED). For the established eating disorders, the central defining feature falls along the dimension of how much you eat—anorexia represents a problem with eating too little and both bulimia and BED represent problems with eating too much. Bulimia has the added feature of behaviors intended to compensate for eating too much that distinguishes it from BED. Purging disorder differs

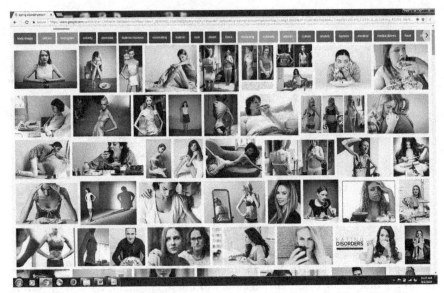

Figure 1.1 Screenshot for results from a search of Google Images for "eating disorder person" demonstrating popular perception that eating disorder means anorexia nervosa and occurs in mostly in young, white, non-Hispanic females.
Credit: Google and the Google logo are registered trademarks of Google LLC, used with permission.

from each of these disorders. Individuals with purging disorder eat neither too little nor too much. If you were dining out with someone with purging disorder (or even able to observe them in the privacy of their homes), their eating wouldn't look different from someone trying to watch their weight, which means they'd look like a lot of people. In purging disorder, the eating disturbance occurs in how that person responds to what they ate. As one woman described, "After I eat a regular meal I feel so disgustingly full that it's just something I 'need' to do." They feel compelled to get rid of food through self-induced vomiting, or through misuse of laxatives, diuretics, or other medications. They purge to avoid gaining weight or becoming fat. Although purging can occur in both anorexia and bulimia, it's not the central feature of either disorder, and both disorders occur in individuals who have never purged.

You wouldn't be able to tell that a person has purging disorder just by looking at them. They eat enough food to maintain a minimally healthy body weight. This distinguishes them from individuals with anorexia, in whom restricted food intake causes medically low body weight. On the outside, people with purging disorder look just like people without eating disorders. As one girl explained, "To all, I appeared to be a healthy, normal girl, but I was secretly destroying my body." Their bodies can range from being somewhat thin to being significantly overweight or even obese, just like the bodies of people without eating disorders.

Individuals with purging disorder don't consume more food than most people eat—distinguishing them from individuals with bulimia and BED, in whom

Do We Need Another Eating Disorder?   5

bingeing involves a loss of control while eating an excessive quantity of food. For example, a person with bulimia or BED might eat an entire package of store-bought cookies and a box of sugary cereal with milk, consuming over 3,000 calories in a single sitting, because they couldn't stop eating until all the food was gone. The average size of binges is approximately 3,600 calories in bulimia and BED, according to feeding lab studies. This represents an abnormally large amount of food that most people would experience as undesirable and unpleasant. Those with purging disorder eat no more food than most people eat, which means less than 1,000 calories in two hours, according to feeding lab studies. If you're wondering how much food goes into 1,000 calories, this could accommodate a blueberry scone and a Matcha Green Tea Frappuccino at Starbucks. However, this is an upper limit. In purging disorder, the average consumption prior to purging is around 500 to 750 calories (meaning people purge after either the blueberry scone *or* the Frappuccino—neither of which is excessive).

Some individuals with purging disorder experience a loss of control over their eating and may even subjectively experience their food intake as large. For example, one woman described how she had eaten an "entire bag of potato chips." With additional probing, she shared that she had gotten the bag from a vending machine. But for her, this single serving represented an enormous amount of food. Another woman's largest out-of-control "binge" involved 40 calories. These perceptions represent distortions of reality and a feature of the illness. However, not all people with purging disorder experience their eating as out of control. Some just need to purge to feel control over the effects of food on their bodies: "We threw up because we ate normally and felt fat, or felt that it would make us fat." So, if purging disorder is not captured by any of the three existing disorders, why aren't there four eating disorders—anorexia, bulimia, BED, and purging disorder?

CREATING A NEW DIAGNOSIS

Creating a new diagnosis means identifying a collection of symptoms or features that appear to go together and negatively impact people. The presence of distress or problems functioning in daily life distinguish a disorder from healthy behavior. For example, if symptoms cause dejection or problems at school, work, or in important relationships, this would be evidence that the condition is harmful and not healthy. Importantly, people do all sorts of harmful and unhealthy things that are not necessarily signs of mental illness. Have you ever crossed the street when the red flashing hand indicated that you should yield the right of way to vehicles that could crush your body? Yes? Repeatedly? Me too. So have most people walking in any semi-urban or urban setting. Even if something can or has been harmful (according to the Governors Highway Safety Association, over 1,500 people were killed crossing intersections in the United States in 2017[2]), that's not enough to make it a mental disorder. To be a mental disorder, the set of behaviors, thoughts, and feelings needs to be relatively rare and unusual, and cannot be considered normative either within the broader culture or within a subculture. Nor can something that a person chooses to do as an act of defiance against society or social norms be considered mental illness. The absence of choice in mental illness can be experienced as an inability to control what's happening or as a compulsion to engage in a behavior. For example, vomiting in purging disorder, food restriction in anorexia, and even hand washing in obsessive-compulsive disorder are intentional. However, no one has chosen to feel compelled to engage in these acts. The key hallmarks that distinguish a mental illness from normality are (1) causing harm, (2) being (relatively) uncommon, and (3) being outside a person's control.

Purging means inducing the forceful evacuation of matter from the body. It purposefully mimics the body's response to a threat. For example, when a virus, bacteria, or poison enters the body, vomiting and diarrhea attempt to rid the body of the infection or toxin. Similarly, excessive urination occurs when the kidneys work to flush out toxins filtered from the bloodstream. As a biological function, vomiting, diarrhea, and excessive urination signify a problem, or threat to the body, and represent the body's attempt to eliminate that problem and restore health. Reflecting this function, the word "purge" means *to purify* according to the Catechism of the Catholic Church.

In Catholicism, purgatory is where souls are cleansed of their sins before entering heaven. Throughout literature, we find examples of purging being used to eliminate moral contamination, such as the final chapter in Aldous Huxley's *Brave New World* in which a Native American character seeks to rid himself of the ills of the modern dystopia by drinking mustard water to induce vomiting. This fictional account was inspired by the real-life Navajo sweet-emetic ritual—a purification rite employed to cure illness of bodily or spiritual origins. For this rite, the afflicted are brought into a special hut and given a basin containing an emetic that they drink to induce vomiting. The vomiting is viewed as central to eliminating pollution to restore bodily and spiritual health. While purging is a sign of malady across these diverse contexts, it is not a sign of mental illness because it has either a medical or cultural basis and is time limited. Purging is not maintained as an ongoing way of life.

Whether purging occurs due to a physical illness, as a cultural practice, or as an eating disorder, it signifies a deviation from what is "right"—a sign that something is wrong—and an attempt to re-establish goodness. In the context of purging disorder, food is viewed as a threat because it contributes to fat, which is experienced as vile and disgusting. People with purging disorder seek to rid their bodies of this threat. Because food is not a toxin or sin but is necessary to survival, the "threat" from food can never be completely eliminated, and purging becomes habitual. Habitual purging is a problem because purging is a violent act. As described in chapter 6, purging exacts an incredible toll on the body, contributing to a host of medical complications. Bodies are not equipped to withstand purging that recurs over weeks, much less months. One man who purged for over 40 years because of concerns about his weight described how over this time "stomach acids have made my teeth, especially the inside of my incisors, smooth." In these ways, purging disorder differs dramatically from the wide range of behaviors that surround normal and healthy eating. However, establishing that deliberately vomiting (or inducing diarrhea or excessive urination) is not healthy or normal does not automatically translate into making purging disorder an official eating disorder. Purging occurs in both anorexia and bulimia, and some have argued that anorexia, bulimia, and purging disorder belong together as a single eating disorder.

Creating a new diagnosis means identifying a collection of symptoms and features that are different from established disorders. Early efforts at diagnostic classification for mental disorders drew from biology and medicine and sought to "carve nature at its joints."[3] More and more, we realize that distinctions we draw may be more functional than natural. A natural distinction is based in nature, like the distinction between dogs and cats. A functional distinction may not reflect any natural or biologically based difference. Instead, it may reflect demographic differences in who is affected by an illness, what treatments work for that illness, and illness course and outcomes. This creates a challenge because it means we employ culturally based values to choose what merits identification whenever we create a diagnosis.

Within the broader mental health field there is an ongoing debate between two camps: lumpers and splitters. Lumpers and splitters differ in their approach to identifying and distinguishing among mental disorders. Lumpers focus on commonalities, while splitters focus on differences. Lumpers would group under one diagnostic category what splitters would divide into separate diagnostic categories. For the lumpers, there is a strong case that mental disorders do not represent unique categories, but all reside along dimensions with one another. From this perspective, purging disorder is not different from other eating disorders in a way that requires its own diagnosis—differences are a matter of degree or severity, and purging disorder falls on a continuum somewhere between what we call anorexia and what we call bulimia (Figure 1.2). Some of my own work suggests that this may be true.

Over time, a person may go from having anorexia to bulimia to purging disorder. Did they really suffer from three different eating disorders or did they have one eating disorder that changed with time? Further, the clear demarcations between anorexia, bulimia, and purging disorder get blurry when we consider the cases that exist between their boundaries. For example, by definition, a patient with anorexia will be underweight, and a patient with purging disorder will not. Between them, however, may be a patient who has lost a great deal of weight but not enough to be underweight and who purges but does not binge. According to the DSM-5, this person could be diagnosed with atypical anorexia nervosa, an otherwise specified feeding or eating disorder (OSFED). Atypical anorexia with purging represents a bridge between purging anorexia and purging disorder, with all three residing on a continuum of current weight and weight loss. Similarly, purging disorder falls on a continuum with purging bulimia according to the amount of food consumed before purging. We have interviewed countless women who purge after eating episodes that fall into a middle ground between diagnoses. They may be eating more than what most people would *probably* eat in a given situation, but it's difficult to determine because people differ a *lot* in how much they comfortably eat. Sure, eating an entire large pizza in an hour is clearly excessive,

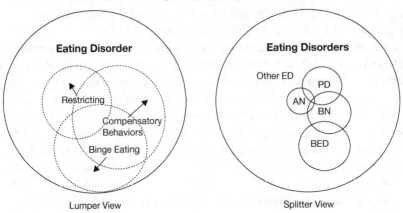

Figure 1.2 View of how eating disorder(s) could be viewed as either one eating disorder or several separate eating disorders. AN = anorexia nervosa; BED = binge-eating disorder; BN = bulimia nervosa; ED = eating disorder; PD = purging disorder.

but is eating all but one slice normal? What about eating half of the pizza in the first hour, waiting a couple of hours and then eating the second half? Ultimately, we don't have a precise threshold for exactly how much pizza is too much pizza to consume in two hours. And that's just pizza. Thresholds get even murkier when you move on to combinations of foods. Purging after eating an amount that is in this "gray zone" (not clearly excessive but also not clearly typical) falls on a continuum between bulimia and purging disorder.

Given these points, it's fair to ask if we really need another eating disorder diagnosis. If there are no objective boundaries to be found in nature, can't we be more parsimonious and make everything just one diagnosis— "eating disorder"? There are brilliant experts in my field who have advocated for exactly this approach. But there are at least two reasons to exercise caution before lumping everything into a single diagnostic category.

First, how do you decide which continuum matters most? Purging disorder could be placed on a continuum with anorexia, if the central feature is weight or weight loss. Or it could be placed on a continuum with bulimia if the central feature is amount of food consumed. But this view starts with the assumption that the central defining feature of the established eating disorder is the only one that matters and ignores the central feature of purging disorder—purging. As noted already, not everyone with anorexia or bulimia purges, and no one with BED purges. Thus, purging disorder resides on a continuum with other eating disorders if we ignore purging or treat purging as incidental. If we start with the central feature of purging disorder—the purging behavior—and ask if this resides on a continuum with anorexia, bulimia, and BED, the answer is no. Inducing purging is not a matter of degree. One does not have a "touch of purging"— a person either purges or they don't. It's binary. And many patients with eating disorders have never purged, creating a clear boundary between purging disorder and every eating disorder in which people don't purge (Figure 1.3). And much of my research has supported this point of discontinuity.

Second, even if we could identify a single continuum (or set of continua) on which all eating disorders reside, there are places along that continuum at which the implications of illness change. For example, if we think about blood pressure, we can easily agree that hypertension and hypotension (blood pressure that is too high and blood pressure that is too low) reside on a continuum with one another. However, the causes of hypertension and hypotension and their treatments differ so dramatically that it is useful to identify them as separate conditions. To my knowledge, no one has proposed a broad category of "blood pressure disorder" that would merge these two together just because they fall on opposite ends of a spectrum. Even for aspects of purging disorder that do reside on a continuum with anorexia (body weight) or bulimia (amount of food consumed), at certain thresholds the factors contributing to and resulting from the severity of symptoms produce functional disparities. Using different names is an effect approach to capture meaningful boundaries between functionally distinct syndromes. These same reasons explain how we got the official eating disorders we have today despite the overlap among them.

Once upon a time, anorexia nervosa was a newly identified disorder, as was bulimia nervosa, and BED—how did each of these achieve that status? For each disorder, a repeating pattern emerged in which a critical mass of evidence pushed each condition from obscurity to widespread recognition, leading to an accepted name and definition. A balance between scientific evidence and sociohistorical context contributed to the recognition and creation of each of the current official eating disorders as "new" eating disorders.

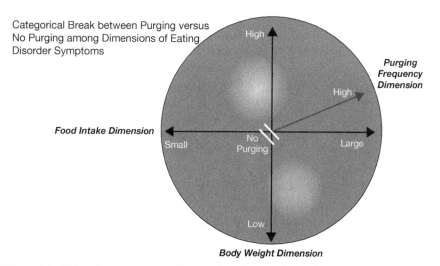

Figure 1.3 Although some aspects of eating disorders reside on dimensions with normality, purging is categorically distinct from normality.

WHEN THE OLD EATING DISORDERS WERE NEW

Anorexia is not only the first eating disorder that comes to mind for people; it's also the first eating disorder that was formally identified and named in the medical literature. Sir William Gull, working in London, introduced the term "anorexia nervosa" to the medical field in 1874 to describe a series of patients, mostly young females, who had started starving themselves for no apparent reason. In a prior lecture given in 1868, Gull made a passing reference to *hysteric apepsia* to describe self-starvation in some patients, but it was really the 1874 case series that garnered attention from the newly forming field of psychiatry. Like the features we see today, patients were indifferent to their own state and quite physically active despite their emaciation. Charles Lasègue, working in Paris, named and described *l'anorexie hysterique* in several of his female patients in 1873. The condition closely mirrored what Gull described and was published a year before Gull's paper, but the name Gull chose rose above the competing terms that were emerging from around the world. Indeed, during the final quarter of the 19th century, physicians from Italy, Russia, Australia, and the United States were describing mysterious cases of girls starving themselves with no medical cause. Moving from the late 19th century into the early 20th century, anorexia was recognized as a rare but serious psychiatric disorder because patients who did not recover were at considerable risk of death from starvation. Even though the diagnosis was included in the first edition of the DSM published in 1952, most psychiatrists never encountered a case outside of textbooks. At that time, anorexia nervosa was listed among a disparate set of disorders because there was no category for eating disorders.

During the latter half of the 20th century, anorexia stopped being an extremely rare condition. The number of new cases seeking treatment was growing larger with each passing year, and programs specifically designed to treat this condition arose. Within these programs, clinicians started seeing patients whose problems resembled anorexia but did not fully match the diagnosis. More than 100 years after Gull introduced anorexia nervosa as a new disorder, Gerald Russell, also working in London, introduced the term "bulimia nervosa" in a 1979 article titled, "Bulimia nervosa: an ominous variant of anorexia nervosa."[4] His report described a series of 30 patients who were not underweight, who were bingeing and purging, and who were terrified of becoming fat. Publication of his article coincided with reports of binge–purge syndromes in normal-weight young women published in German and Spanish and concerns that bulimia or bulimarexia had become an epidemic on college campuses, affecting up to 15% of college women. Within a year, in 1980, bulimia became an official disorder included next to anorexia nervosa in the DSM-III, among disorders usually first evident in infancy, childhood, or adolescence.

For both anorexia and bulimia, there seemed to be a rapid shift in recognition in which experts from around the world began naming a condition that they were encountering too often to ignore and that was too different to be folded into existing diagnostic categories. Terms used to describe the conditions varied by author, with each choosing names they felt best captured the nature of the illness. In addition, some features varied across their descriptions. Like Gull's and Lasègue's descriptions of anorexia nervosa, several authors described a self-starvation disorder in young women. But neither Gull's nor Lasègue's patients expressed concerns about weight or shape—just a mortal fear of eating—while one of their contemporaries noted that his patient refused to eat to ensure that she could fit a ribbon around her waist because she didn't want to become fat like her mother. Like Russell's description of bulimia nervosa, bulimia in the DSM-III involved large out-of-control binges. But unlike Russell's bulimia nervosa, DSM-III bulimia did not necessarily involve purging or compensatory behavior or body image concerns and was so broadly defined that it could accommodate cases of bulimia and BED. Indeed, some of the early literature on BED referred to it as "nonpurging bulimia" to distinguish it from most work conducted in those who binged and vomited. This changed after the 1987 publication of the DSM-III-R, in which bulimia was renamed "bulimia nervosa" and was defined by bingeing, compensatory behaviors (which included but extended beyond purging), and preoccupation with weight and shape.

BED had a less meteoric rise in recognition, potentially because it was absorbed in the original DSM-III definition of bulimia, potentially because it lacks the alarming features of emaciation or purging that differ so much from normal eating. Albert Stunkard, working in Philadelphia, named this condition in 1959, describing it in a subset of patients seeking weight loss for obesity. These patients had recurrent binge episodes, didn't compensate, and differed demographically from the majority of those with anorexia—Stunkard's patients were older, middle-aged individuals and far more of them were men. But very little additional work was completed on BED.[5]

The lack of work on BED changed when Robert Spitzer, who had served as the editor for the DSM-III and DSM-III-R, advocated for the inclusion of BED as a new eating disorder in the DSM-IV. Allen Frances, editor for the DSM-IV, resisted this proposal and expressed concern regarding over-pathologizing the common occurrence of overeating. Ultimately, a team of five eating disorder researchers, referred to as the DSM-IV Eating Disorders Workgroup,[6] would examine the case for BED's inclusion. In a published transcript of the DSM-IV workgroup's deliberations, Dr. Frances commented, "It's the proliferation problem. *DSM-III-R* has twice as many disorders as *DSM-II*. If this continues the system will become so cumbersome it'll be unusable. In *DSM-III* and *DSM-III-R*, if a diagnosis was interesting and there was desire to stimulate research, it was put in. For *DSM-IV*, we've made a much higher threshold."[7] Additional concerns included the political ramifications of stigmatizing a segment of the obese population, that the disorder would be too common, that BED might not be distinct from bulimia, and that a premature definition of an understudied condition would result in it being accepted as true—the problem of reification. Reification of any diagnosis as "true" before enough evidence was collected could make it difficult to change, improve, or eliminate an invalid one. It seemed unlikely that enough evidence could be collected to support BED's inclusion. In fact, at the time of the first discussion, it was unclear if there was enough time to even explore the *option* of its inclusion.

Ultimately,[8] the compromise in 1994 was to include BED in the DSM-IV as a provisional diagnosis in the broad, heterogeneous category of eating disorder not otherwise specified (EDNOS). Proposed diagnostic criteria were placed in the manual's appendix. Another change to the DSM-IV was that the two official eating disorders, anorexia nervosa and bulimia nervosa, appeared in their own chapter, titled "Eating Disorders."

The May 2013 publication of the DSM-5 introduced BED as an official eating disorder of equal standing with anorexia and bulimia. A search for "binge eating disorder" in the American Psychological Association's PsychINFO database yielded 840 papers published between 1959 and May 2013, with 825 published since BED's inclusion in the DSM-IV. The wealth of information that came from this work supported including BED as a new disorder in the DSM-5. This reveals an important relationship between scientific evidence and recognition of a new disorder. As pressures mounted to ensure that disorders met stringent criteria for inclusion in the DSM, the evidence required for admission increased exponentially across editions. Yet, the likelihood of obtaining that evidence is exponentially enhanced by including the disorder in the DSM (Figure 1.4). Returning to the DSM-IV workgroup's early deliberations on BED, the following exchange[9] highlights this dilemma clearly.

> Walsh: The work group agrees these people [with BED] are out there.
> Mitchell: But 18 months is quick. It's taken us 10 years to nail down Bulimia.
> Spitzer: Yes, it was my wisdom to include Bulimia in 1980 when it was new—like BED is now. That led to a decade of research which has helped us define it.

We Study What We Define

Easy Search	Advanced Search	Citation Finder	Cited
#	Query	Databases	Results
1. ☐	("binge eating disorder"):Any Field and	PsycINFO ,	840
2. ☐	("binge eating disorder"):Any Field and [1994	PsycINFO ,	825

Figure 1.4 "We study what we define:" Search results for articles published on binge-eating disorder prior to its inclusion in the DSM-5 and the number published after its inclusion as a named and defined disorder in the DSM-IV. Only 15 papers were published before the DSM-IV and 825 were published after 1994, even though binge-eating disorder was first named in 1959.

Credit: The PsycINFO® Database screenshot is reproduced with permission of the American Psychological Association, publisher of the PsycINFO® database, all rights reserved. Search initiated May 2013.

However, despite the incredible volume of research conducted prior to BED's inclusion in the DSM-5, its official recognition was not free of controversy. In a *Psychology Today* blog, Dr. Frances ranked BED fifth in a list of the "ten worst changes" in the DSM-5 that should be ignored, writing, "5) Excessive eating 12 times in 3 months is no longer just a manifestation of gluttony and the easy availability of really great tasting food. DSM 5 has instead turned it into a psychiatric illness called Binge Eating Disorder."[10] In this blog and in interviews, Dr. Frances noted concerns about profit-related motivations for the publisher of the DSM and for pharmaceutical companies given an ever-expanding number of "patients" (a.k.a., customers). This response highlights the implications of creating a new disorder and the sociohistorical context within which purging disorder's potential to become a new disorder is being weighed.

In some ways, purging disorder can be thought of as the inverse of BED. Individuals with BED binge but do not purge; individuals with purging disorder purge but do not binge. Between the two of them, purging is clearly more distinct from normality. Some of my favorite quotes from the ethnography on the DSM-IV workgroup's deliberations would be profoundly disturbing if Dr. Frances's comments referred to purging disorder instead of BED. These include Dr. Frances telling Dr. Spitzer, "I like your diagnosis. In fact, at times, I even have your diagnosis."[11] And later asking, "Are you testing for prevalence in your field trial? That's a serious, serious problem. You've got to demonstrate that this diagnosis isn't present in 50% of college girls."[12] Purging is such an alarming behavior that it's unlikely Dr. Frances would casually joke about having purging disorder. Further, if 50% of college women were purging on a regular basis, we would see large-scale public health initiatives to address the problem rather than concluding that it wasn't really that big of a deal. So, why wasn't purging disorder included in the DSM-IV? Because no one had identified it; no one had even given it a name when decisions were being made for the DSM-IV.

NAMING PURGING DISORDER IN THE MEDICAL LITERATURE

In 2005, I used the term "purging disorder" to describe women who were purging by self-induced vomiting, laxatives, or diuretics after consuming normal or small amounts of food to control their weight or shape. The title of the article, "Purging disorder: an ominous variant of bulimia nervosa?" was an homage to Russell's paper on bulimia. I ended the title with a question mark because I understood how much more work would be needed before any conclusion could be drawn. I set out to name and describe a collection of symptoms and features that hung together and affected individuals in a particular way that seemed different from bulimia. Before this article, I wrote another published in 2001 but referred to the condition as "subjective bulimia nervosa." And even before the 2001 article this clinical presentation had been described in a 1986 article written to inform the DSM-III-R workgroup's examples of atypical eating disorders. But it had no name other than "atypical eating disorder group 1," and the fourth example for an EDNOS in the DSM-IV (literally, EDNOS type 4). From 2001 to 2005, I stopped using "subjective bulimia nervosa" when I presented findings at conferences because I realized that name implied that purging disorder was a type of bulimia nervosa, which was looking less and less true according to my data. In addition, by doing this, I excluded from recognition those who purged without ever feeling a loss of control over their eating. Similar to the historical contexts in which anorexia and bulimia gained widespread recognition, reports of purging disorder started appearing from around the world, with cases in Italy, Australia, England, Germany, and Japan. Shortly after entering the 21st century, the field was encountering alarmingly high numbers of women who purged without bingeing and were not underweight—women with an eating disorder that did not fit into anorexia, bulimia, or BED diagnoses.

In the leadup to the DSM-5, the *International Journal of Eating Disorders* published special issues focused on the classification of eating disorder diagnoses in 2007 and 2009, and I was invited to contribute reviews of purging disorder to both. The 2007 article identified 10 empirical (data-based) papers, across which seven different names had been used in reference to the condition, including "subjective bulimia nervosa," "EDNOS-P," "purge eating disorder," and "purging disorder." Definitions differed across these papers, and even papers using the same name had somewhat different definitions, with "purging" sometimes being expanded to include fasting and excessive exercise. (For the record, fasting and excessive or compulsive exercise are compensatory behaviors that may be used in bulimia, but they are not actually purging behaviors because they do not involve forceful evacuation of matter from the body.) By the 2009 review, another 20 empirical papers had been published, reflecting a tripling of the scientific work on the topic. In contrast to the use of "purging disorder" in only 1 of the first 10 articles published on the condition (my 2005 article), "purging disorder" was used in 7 of the last 10 articles published (definitely not all mine). In addition to greater consistency in terminology, there was greater consistency in definitions.

Key conclusions of the 2009 review were organized around established criteria for considering a new diagnosis:

> *Criterion 1. Is There Ample Literature on Purging Disorder?* With 48 total
> publications on purging disorder, including 30 empirical papers (6 from
> my lab and 24 from other researchers), there was ample literature on
> purging disorder. It wasn't BED's 840 publications as of May 2013, but it
> was considerably more than BED's 15 publications as of 1994.
>
> *Criterion 2. Is There a Common Set of Diagnostic Criteria for Purging
> Disorder and Are There Assessment Tools Available for Measuring the
> Syndrome?* Although this was clearly absent in the 2007 review, the
> definition of purging disorder had largely coalesced across more
> recent studies. Multiple groups were identifying purging disorder in
> those who purged without bingeing and who were not underweight.
> Further, the "gold standard" for eating disorders assessment, the *Eating*

Disorders Examination, was ideally suited to identifying the disorder, distinguishing it from anorexia and bulimia, and capturing its severity and remission status.

Criterion 3. Is There Diagnostic Reliability? There was. People tend to be very clear on what the definition of purging is. There is high agreement among different interviewers about the presence or absence of purging, and high agreement over time in people's own reports of whether or not they had purged.

Criterion 4. Can Purging Disorder be Differentiated from Other Eating Disorders (and Normality)? Here the literature had some important gaps. While every single study ever published supported that purging disorder was, indeed, not normal and was clearly a clinically significant disorder of eating, comparisons between purging disorder and other eating disorders were a bit sparse. All my research had compared purging disorder to bulimia—reflecting my early bias in thinking of it as a variant of bulimia. Unfortunately, a lot of the field followed suit, and very few studies compared purging disorder to anorexia or BED. That was true then, and it is less true now. But the biggest challenge in identifying this new disorder was determining whether it should be distinguished from the existing eating disorders or whether the definition of existing eating disorders should be expanded to include purging disorder. Indeed, the International Classification of Diseases published its 11th edition in June 2018, and it redefined a binge-eating episode as "a distinct period of time during which the individual experiences a subjective loss of control over eating, eating notably more or differently than usual, and feels unable to stop eating or limit the type or amount of food eaten."[13] Those who purge after feeling a loss of control over their eating could be diagnosed with bulimia using ICD-11 criteria even if they didn't eat that much. That revision subsumes many individuals with purging disorder into a diagnosis of bulimia. Importantly, given that many patients purge without ever feeling a loss of control over their eating, it doesn't account for all cases of purging disorder.

Criterion 5. Is There Syndrome Validity? For this article, we focused on a specific kind of validity—the extent to which a diagnosis helped clinicians know how to treat the illness and patients' likelihood of recovery. Again, at the time of the 2009 review, considerable data supported that purging disorder looked different from bulimia on several factors, but there were limited data on course, treatment response, and outcome. These are all indicators of clinical utility, or the value of the diagnosis in a treatment setting—a key criterion for adding a diagnosis to the DSM-5.

We ended the review by discussing the pros and cons of four options for addressing purging disorder in the DSM-5. Option 1 was to do nothing—leave purging disorder as an unnamed example in a heterogenous group of eating disorders that just weren't quite anorexia or bulimia. The pro was that this option certainly minimized proliferation of diagnoses and would not contribute to a diagnostic system that was unweildy or untrustworthy. However, it was already clear that purging disorder was a clinically significant problem that had been buried in a heterogenous group for which little to no useful information was being systematically obtained. For example, the largest and most representative epidemiological study of mental disorders conducted in the United States at the time couldn't estimate how many people had purging disorder because participants were only asked about purging if they binged. For those who didn't binge, all questions about purging were skipped. Fortunately, epidemiological data from *other* countries made clear the large number of people who would be ignored by doing nothing. Ultimately, we noted that doing nothing would limit collection of needed information to validate the disorder and to help the considerable number of people currently suffering it.

Option 2 was to redefine diagnostic criteria for official eating disorders to absorb purging disorder. The pros were that it minimized proliferation of diagnoses *and* it would support insurance coverage for treatment of those purging after eating normal amounts of food, even though they weren't underweight and weren't bingeing. The cons were that no revision to existing diagnostic criteria could accommodate all cases of purging disorder without damaging the clinical utility of anorexia or bulimia. The only way to include all cases of purging disorder in the definition of bulimia was to eliminate the binge-eating criterion. However, comparisons between purging disorder and bulimia showed significant differences on psychological and biological factors that might have major implications for treatment. The only way to include all cases of purging disorder in the definition of anorexia was to eliminate the low-weight criterion for anorexia. Although there weren't many studies comparing purging disorder to anorexia, too much evidence supported the low-weight criterion for anorexia to change this aspect of its definition. Even if purging disorder could be absorbed into one of these diagnostic categories without impacting their clinical utility, there wasn't enough evidence to determine whether it should go into a broader category for bulimia or a broader category for anorexia.

Option 3 was to include purging disorder as an official eating disorder diagnosis—give it a name, diagnostic criteria, and a diagnostic code, putting it on equal footing with anorexia and bulimia. The pro was that this would support insurance coverage for treatment and promote research into the causes and consequences of the illness, which could ultimately lead to the prevention and treatment of purging disorder. The clear con was this meant creating a new eating disorder diagnosis before sufficient scientific evidence supported the decision. Further, once the diagnostic criteria were specified, all research on purging disorder would use those criteria—whether they accurately defined the disorder or not. This is the problem of reification raised during deliberations on the inclusion of BED in the DSM-IV.

Option 4 was to include purging disorder as a named condition with a provisional definition. This represented a compromise between Option 1 and Option 3 that maximized the benefits while minimizing the costs of each of those extremes. This option offered an opportunity for researchers to "study what we define" without setting in stone a definition that requires further investigation. Future editions of the DSM would need scientific study of purging disorder. And the first step in the scientific study of anything is to form the hypothesis that it exists. No field of science has gained much ground by accepting the null hypothesis that there is no difference between groups without ever testing it—this is the classic fallacy of equating an absence of evidence with evidence of an absence. A name and provisional definition would pave the way for tests of whether or not there were differences between purging disorder and anorexia, bulimia, and other eating disorders in terms of course, outcome, and treatment response. Such research would be enormously helpful to those suffering from purging disorder. In addition to these academic and practical benefits, this approach mitigated long-noted problems with prematurely introducing disorders in the absence of evidence supporting their clinical utility. Purging disorder would not be an official diagnosis and would not add to the overall number of diagnoses in the DSM-5. The final advantage of this option is that it allowed the needs of those currently suffering from purging disorder to be recognized.

One person wrote, "From my experience, I have always felt like a failed bulimic, but not quite an anorexic [. . .] like a grey area that doesn't fit." Another: "I have always thought that I fell out of the Bulimia and Anorexia 'guidelines' and that was a good excuse to tell myself I probably did not have a 'disorder.'" "Every time I try to get help, the doctors will refer to my habits as binging and purging, and even when I explain otherwise I see them write binging on their papers [. . .] Over the past 4 months (after I started throwing up blood) I have been coming to terms with my disorder, and seeking treatment, but have had very little luck with finding someone willing to get past their preconceptions and stop assigning me symptoms that I don't have." Or "Many people feel that if you do not meet the DSM description, you do not have an eating disorder [. . .] I began to purge, but I did not binge. But because I was never underweight, not many noticed that I had a problem. I did at one point go see a counselor to have an intake, who at the end of the session basically told me I was fine." Or even under the best circumstances, "When I was diagnosed in [. . .] I was told I had an 'eating-disorder-otherwise-unspecified' or something along those lines. It was oddly frustrating to hear I did not meet the requirements for bulimia. I had come to a point where I realized I needed help, had accepted I had a problem and found it hard to hear that my problem didn't have a name."

The 2009 review was commissioned by the DSM-5 workgroup, and we were asked not to express a preference for any of the options. After the review was completed, new studies might be published that would influence the final decision in ways that could not be predicted. Thus, any recommendations might be premature or viewed as biasing decisions that needed to be made within the structure of the DSM's organization and process. This process was established to ensure consistency and rigor for all diagnoses under consideration—not just those in the eating disorders section. Of course, it was unlikely that information on long-term course and treatment response would emerge with so little time left before the fifth edition was scheduled for publication, and nothing earth-shattering appeared on purging disorder before the DSM-5 workgroup's deliberations were completed. Thus, Option 4 continued to have the most benefits and the fewest costs, and Option 4 is largely what happened.

Purging disorder is a named condition in the DSM-5. It falls within the broad category OSFED, much as BED appeared as a named condition in the DSM-IV's EDNOS. As a set, the disorders classified as OSFED do not have the same standing as anorexia, bulimia, or BED. Each of those eating disorders possesses its own diagnostic criteria, diagnostic code, and subsection of the chapter on feeding and eating disorders describing diagnostic features, associated features, prevalence, development and course, risk and prognostic factors, culture-related diagnostic issues (gender-related diagnostic issues), diagnostic markers, suicide risk, functional consequences, differential diagnosis, and comorbidity. The DSM-5 offers the following description for the newly named condition: "Purging disorder: Recurrent purging behavior to influence weight or shape (e.g., self-induced vomiting; misuse of laxatives, diuretics, or other medications) in the absence of binge eating."[14] No additional information is provided because purging disorder is not a separate, official eating disorder like anorexia, bulimia, or BED. Its diagnostic code is the same as that for atypical anorexia nervosa and night eating syndrome (NES)—although it shares no overlapping features with NES and does not even seem to reside on any identifiable continuum with this fellow OSFED.

Provisional diagnostic criteria were not provided for any of the OSFEDs in the DSM-5. This decision reflected the consequences of including provisional diagnostic criteria for BED in the DSM-IV. Revising BED's criteria based on research was nearly impossible. Almost all studies of BED had used the provisional criteria in selecting participants. This fulfilled funding agencies' expectations that methods could be reproduced across studies and contributed to the accumulation of a wealth of information on BED's course, outcome, and treatment. But it also represented the problem of reification because we only had data on BED as it had been defined in the DSM-IV. In contrast, the descriptions for OSFEDs in the DSM-5 provide enough information to ensure some consistency across studies, do not preclude variations across studies that could be used to refine the definition, and largely follow what the field was already doing.

Although purging disorder is not an official eating disorder in the DSM-5, it is a specified eating disorder. Ultimately, Dr. Frances's point about proliferation is right—there has to be a limit to the number of disorders that get named. If everything that is different from normal eating could be a disorder, then there would be an eating disorder for those who repeatedly chew and spit out their food without swallowing it, and one for those who follow strict rules about eating clean or correctly, referred to as orthorexia, and so on and so forth. To address this practical limit, the DSM-5 includes a broad "unspecified eating disorder" option that captures everything that merits diagnosis but has garnered insufficient evidence to be included as either an official eating disorder or as an OSFED.

WHY WE NEED PURGING DISORDER

In the fairy tale "Rumpelstiltskin," the Miller's Daughter must name the man who has spun straw into gold in order to keep her son—reflecting a long-held superstition that the very act of naming an entity gives one power over that entity. The cultural belief that names have power is evident in the modern practice of diagnosis in which patients feel reassured when their collection of symptoms and signs has a name, even when the name provides little more than a shorthand reference for their described experiences. Naming creates the feeling that something is real, that one is not alone in having experienced the condition, and that there is hope for a good outcome. As one person wrote, "Finally a name for what is wrong with me. When you don't fit into either category of eating disorders, no one can help you. I just wanted to say I'm glad you have found a name for the demon that haunts me." The key challenge is that the process of naming provides so much reassurance that it can be difficult to relinquish names that do not work toward their ultimate goals—the goal of controlling mental illness through effective prevention and treatment.

The inclusion of purging disorder as a named and described condition in the DSM-5 has motivated considerable work. We now know much more about its development and course, risk and prognostic factors, consequences, and treatment. And what we've learned supports that purging disorder merits recognition as a new eating disorder. Based on what happened following the inclusion of bulimia in the DSM-III and BED in the DSM-IV, we can expect this body of research to continue to grow as we head toward the next edition of the DSM, the DSM 5.1. So, yes, we need another eating disorder. And, in the rest of this book, I want to share with you what we've been able to learn about this new eating disorder.

Who, When, and Where?

The Social, Historical, and Cultural Context of Purging Disorder

"New diseases are rare, and a disease that selectively befalls the young, rich, and beautiful is practically unheard of."[1] This was the opening of Hilde Bruch's seminal book on anorexia, *The Golden Cage*. The legacy of her description is reflected in the collection of powerful Google images depicting eating disorders in mostly young white females (see Figure 1.1). But is this true for purging disorder? Not exactly.[2]

WHO SUFFERS FROM PURGING DISORDER?

Most studies of purging disorder have excluded males as if the disorder doesn't impact them, but that's absolutely incorrect. Purging disorder does impact males but is more likely to affect women and girls. In a study of U.S. college students, women were nine times more likely than men to suffer from purging disorder. And studies of teens in the United States, Canada, Germany, and Australia found that purging disorder was about two to five times more likely to affect girls than boys. Combining estimates across studies, roughly 1 in 40 women and girls have purging disorder right now compared to 1 in 200 males.

Percentages like 2.5% of females and 0.5% of males may seem small. And they should. By definition, a disorder can't be ordinary. But when a small percentage gets multiplied by a large number—like the 84 million U.S. females between the ages of 10 and 49, this translates into more than 2 million women and girls currently suffering from purging disorder, with almost half a million men and boys joining them. In a study following girls from the age of 13 to 20 years, the authors found 447 new cases of purging disorder per 100,000 females per year. By comparison, breast cancer is the most common form of cancer in women, and we see 124.8 new cases of breast cancer per 100,000 females per year, according to the

Centers for Disease Control and Prevention.[3] All of a sudden, the numbers for purging disorder don't seem so small.

Up to 1 in 20 women have had purging disorder at some point in their lives. That last statistic isn't even small. To appreciate just how many women this is, count up the number of women you pass the next time you're walking through a store or down a street; see how quickly you reach 20. Odds are good that one of them had purging disorder at some point in her life. Maybe she has it right now. And if you are the person with purging disorder, all you have to do is keep counting. Because, I promise, you are not alone.

In every single study that has included both genders, purging disorder is more common in females than in males. Why? The answer probably seems obvious— purging to control weight is related to a desire to be thin, and thinness is an ideal of feminine beauty. But I want to consider another possibility: Purging disorder may be more common in females because I only looked at women when I was defining the disorder. The eating disorder treatment program at Massachusetts General Hospital wasn't restricted to women, but among those with eating disorders, women are much more likely than men to seek treatment. So, the purging disorder patients I saw—in fact, *all* of the eating disorder patients I saw—were women. Similarly, that study I was running to compare bulimia and binge-eating disorder (BED)[4] wasn't restricted to women, but women are also significantly more likely to volunteer for research, so the vast majority of callers were female. This means that even as I was trying to understand what purging disorder was, I was looking at it through the lens of who sought treatment and who volunteered for research—women. This approach may have introduced bias into my definition of the illness by focusing on features that reflected the subjects' gender rather than the illness itself.

Dr. Alison Field, professor and chair of Brown University's Department of Epidemiology, studied eating disorders in adolescent girls and boys, following them from when they were 9 years old to when they were 26 years old. From the age of 13 on, around 1 in 50 girls had purging disorder. There were also a handful of boys with purging disorder—using vomiting or laxatives to control their weight without bingeing or being underweight. But a much larger number of boys, 1 in 13, were doing what the authors called "the male equivalent of purging disorder."[5] Similar to all girls and boys with purging disorder, they weren't underweight and they weren't bingeing. But instead of being afraid of gaining weight, these boys were preoccupied with wanting to have bigger, more toned and defined muscles, and they were using dangerous substances to achieve this ideal. If the definition of purging disorder were expanded to include the use of any medications (laxatives, diuretics, anabolic steroids, creatinine) to influence weight or shape, regardless of whether use was in pursuit of thinness or muscularity, then we would see a lot more purging disorder in boys and men. The take-home point is that purging disorder can and does occur in males— and even more of them may experience a variant of purging disorder that currently falls just beyond the boundaries of how we define the illness. Returning to a point made in Chapter 1, the absence of provisional diagnostic criteria for purging disorder in the DSM-5 permits research exploring definitions that may include more boys and men.

Just as most studies have focused on females, most studies have examined adolescents and young adults. In the very small number of studies that included girls younger than 10 years of age, purging disorder has been found, but it is very rare. Risk for developing purging disorder increases around 14 years of age—just as young teens are navigating dramatic physical, emotional, and social changes, so purging disorder does usually begin in early to mid-adolescence. But purging disorder is also present in older individuals. Studies with adult women ranging up to the early to mid-40s show just as many women with purging disorder as do studies focused on younger women. If purging disorder were restricted to teenagers and young adults, then overall percentages should be lower when samples include older women, but they aren't. We don't know whether older women with purging disorder developed it in their teens and never got better or if they developed purging disorder later in life. We do know that purging disorder occurs across the lifespan from adolescence to at least midlife.

With regard to race and ethnicity, no study has supported any association between being white and likelihood of having purging disorder. Across all of our studies, women with purging disorder largely resemble the broader U.S. population in terms of race and ethnicity. Specifically, we have interviewed white, non-Hispanic women, Hispanic women, African-American women, Asian women, and women of more than one race who have purging disorder. A study of urban inner-city youth in the United Kingdom found that 50% of purging disorder cases occurred in non-white females. This underscores the idea that like all eating disorders, purging disorder does not discriminate on the basis of race or ethnicity.

So, if a Google Image search accurately depicted who suffers from purging disorder, we would see more women than men—true. But we would see more men, and ages would span from younger adolescence to middle age. And the images would include people from the full range of racial and ethnic backgrounds that make up the general population.

Returning to Bruch's quote from the beginning of this chapter, another common misconception is that eating disorders are new. Clearly, as we learned in the previous chapter, anorexia and bulimia are not new. But is purging disorder? Of course the disorder had to exist before I could identify and name it. But how long did it exist before it was recognized? Have recent societal and cultural shifts created an eating disorder that hadn't existed before?

Two studies examined purging disorder in the decades leading up to its recognition in successive groups of U.S. college students, beginning in 1982 and extending to the early 2000s. In both, the percentage of college women affected by purging disorder was stable over that period. This means that whatever contributed to the emergence of purging disorder was present more than two decades before I gave it a name. Importantly, we don't have information predating 1982, so these studies can't tell us if purging disorder was just as common in the 1950s, the 1920s, or the late 1800s. But understanding that purging disorder affected 1.6% of college women in 1982—an estimate that's in line with what we see today—forces us to acknowledge that many young women were having this problem long before we started taking notice of it. But how far back into history does purging disorder go?

HISTORICAL ACCOUNTS OF PURGING AND DISORDERS OF PURGING

As near as we can tell, the basic behaviors of the eating disorders, including purging, have existed for centuries. Accounts of self-starvation syndromes that predominantly affected girls and young women date back to the fourth century A.D. As one of the seven deadly sins, gluttony has also existed for centuries, as have accounts of individuals uncontrollably consuming huge quantities of food. Finally, reports of self-induced vomiting are sprinkled throughout historical cases of eating and other disorders.

Some of the most extensive historical accounts of eating pathology exist for medieval saints of the Catholic Church. Among these cases, both St. Catherine of Siena and St. Veronica engaged in self-induced vomiting. St. Catherine used a stalk of fennel to make herself vomit, and St. Veronica would vomit after consuming large quantities of food from her convent's larder. However, the eating behaviors of both women drew attention because of their emaciation and the deliberate nature of their self-starvation. They were among a small number of Catholic nuns in Italy in whom extreme religious fasting moved their confessors to fear their charges' lives would end in sin—specifically, the sin of suicide by starvation. This supports an interpretation that purging occurred in the context of anorexia rather than purging disorder.

Purging among those who were not underweight is described in writings dating from the Roman Empire, with detailed accounts of vomiting by the emperors Claudius (A.D. 41–54) and Vitellius (A.D. 69). However, these and other cases like them resemble bulimia. The records describe gluttonous feasts by mostly older men who had achieved a station in life that afforded them access to large quantities of food, and some of them induced vomiting to continue feasting. Roman philosopher Seneca (4 B.C.–A.D. 65), author of the play *Oedipus*, wrote, "*vomunt ut edant, edunt ut vomant*" ("they vomit that they may eat, they eat that they may vomit").[6] Similar to historical reports of self-induced vomiting in medieval saints, the vomiting was clearly deliberate, but it also followed excessive food intake. Whether or not we can conclude that these Roman emperors had bulimia, it's clear that they didn't have purging disorder. Instead, purging in these and other historical cases followed consumption of unusually large quantities of food.

Did anyone purge without binge eating and without being underweight? The answer seems to be a qualified "yes." A report of patients from the 19th century, around the time that anorexia was first recognized, suggested that there were other girls and young women who "ate well," were not underweight, but vomited everything they consumed. At that time, they were considered cases of *hysteria*—a psychosomatic condition in which emotional distress was expressed as a range of physical illnesses, with blindness, paralysis, and other pseudo-neurological symptoms being most common. These ailments, like eating disorders today, most often afflicted late adolescent and young adult women, which is how hysteria came to be named after the Greek word for the uterus.

In contrast to the minimal attention paid to purging disorder until the turn of the 21st century, "hysterical vomiting" attracted a great deal of attention toward the end of the 1800s. Even before anorexia nervosa was named by Sir William Gull, Dr. Hyde Salter described hysterical vomiting in two young women, ages 19 and 17, in 1868 (Figure 2.1). To distinguish vomiting due to physical conditions—ranging from infection, poison, concussion, and pregnancy—Dr. Salter walked through the evidence that his patients' vomiting was due to a mental condition. For example, in the case of Eliza T., vomiting never occurred in front of a stranger. C.B. could keep down fruit, nuts, oysters, bran biscuits, toast, and tea but would vomit meat, milk, bread, pastry, and vegetables. A further detail on C.B. was given by her sister, who confided that C.B. would steal food to eat in secret and would be able to keep that food down. These sound like eating disorders. Although both girls experienced the vomiting as involuntary, evidence suggests they had some control over the behavior. In addition, both girls vomited after eating normal amounts of food and neither girl was underweight.

Bridget S., described by Dr. Coupland in 1881, was a 24-year-old, unmarried domestic servant, described as "stout, and flabby," who had been in relatively good health before she started vomiting. Like other patients, she reported stomach pain and was initially treated as if she had a gastric ulcer. However, she didn't respond to this or any other treatment, including morphine injections, ice packs to her stomach, and rectal nutrition. Ultimately, she was "cured" by a diet of fish, beef-tea, milk, and an egg, later supplemented with custard-pudding. The initial duration of Bridget S.'s illness rules out causes such as the flu or food poisoning and its response to behavioral treatment supports that it was likely a form of mental illness.

Finally, Dr. Tuckwell described "vomiting of habit" in three patients in 1873.[7] Whereas Dr. Salter held a very pessimistic view of treatment success, Dr. Tuckwell described a simple program in which he interrupted vomiting by observing the physical positioning of patients when they vomited and repositioning them after they ate and waiting until the urge to vomit passed. In all three patients, this treatment cured their vomiting. In Chapter 8, I'll return to certain aspects of

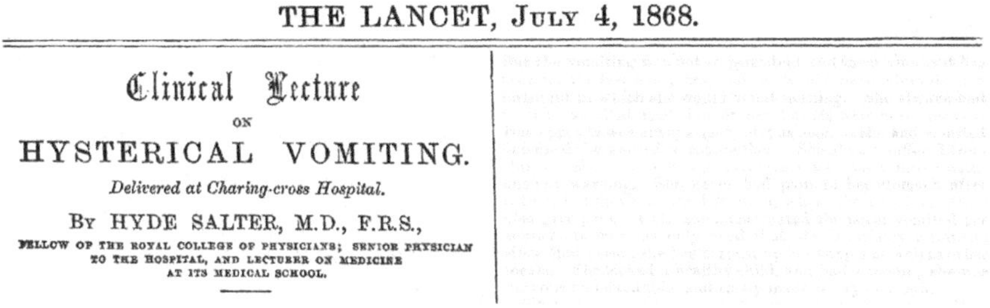

THE LANCET, July 4, 1868.

Clinical Lecture
on
HYSTERICAL VOMITING.
Delivered at Charing-cross Hospital.
By HYDE SALTER, M.D., F.R.S.,
FELLOW OF THE ROYAL COLLEGE OF PHYSICIANS; SENIOR PHYSICIAN
TO THE HOSPITAL, AND LECTURER ON MEDICINE
AT ITS MEDICAL SCHOOL.

Figure 2.1 Published lecture from the late 19th century on cases of hysterical vomiting that reveals similarities and differences from cases of purging disorder today.

Dr. Tuckwell's approach that mimic modern behavioral exposure and response prevention.

Reading through these accounts, I see similarities and differences from purging disorder. Both then and now, vomiting stems from a mental illness surrounding food intake. The vomiting exists in individuals of normal weight who are not bingeing. And the preponderance of hysterical vomiting in adolescent and young adult females is striking. Patients with hysterical vomiting experienced a normal amount of food as being too much, and this matches my own findings in purging disorder. In media coverage of my early research, one finding that attracted a strong response was my description of how individuals with purging disorder felt excessively full, sometimes to the point of nausea and stomachache, after consuming a normal amount of food. One woman wrote, "I never went through the big binging [sic] episodes . . . it was more that I would eat; feel bloated and I would purge to make myself feel relief." Another wrote, "I don't binge, so I never thought I had bulimia. I started feeling really nauseated after eating, and throwing up made me feel better and in my eyes look better." Another woman wrote, "I do not do it because of 'cultural issues with being fat', rather when I eat, it seems that I feel REALLY uncomfortable even when I do not eat very much. [. . .] when I get that uncomfortable feeling, the only thing I can do is purge or I feel like I cannot even breathe sometimes." The parallel between her experience in the 21st century and those of cases in the late 1800s supports a strong connection between what we call purging disorder today and what we called hysterical vomiting back then. My own research (described further in chapter 5) supports biological differences in response to food for women with purging disorder that could cause their increased stomach discomfort. This physiological disruption could explain susceptibility to vomiting after the consumption of normal amounts of food both now and in the late 1800s.

And yet there are differences. Even though there was some evidence that patients with hysteria had some control over vomiting, they experienced their vomiting as an ailment, didn't openly acknowledge their ability to stop vomiting, and didn't hide their vomiting from others.[8] While all of the case reports on hysterical vomiting included information on the patient's weight, ranging from thin to stout, they didn't include any information on the patient's body *image*. Of note, this matches the absence of such information in Gull's and Lasègue's patients with anorexia. Specifically, there was no recording of a fear of fat or a desire to be thin among patients with anorexia or with hysterical vomiting in the late 1800s. In contrast to this absence of information on body image, there was a *plethora* of details on physical complaints—some of which, like excessive thirst, chest discomfort, and lethargy, may be consequences of severe and recurrent vomiting (see chapter 6 for a discussion of the medical consequence of purging). But some of the physical symptoms are just mysterious, even to the treating physician—such as "anomalous irregular pains in parts of the body."[9] Then again, how much of this was shaped by what physicians were looking for then versus what we ask now? I had one father describe the signs that his daughter had been purging in secret (which he and his wife had missed)—trips to the bathroom during meals, dental problems attributed to drinking too much soda when she didn't drink soda, and "recurrent numbness in her legs." The last one stood out because it's exactly the kind of pseudo-neurological symptom that characterizes hysteria, including cases of hysterical vomiting. I've never asked a patient or participant about these kinds of symptoms because they aren't part of how we understand or define eating disorders today. Frankly, I don't know what would happen if I asked someone with purging disorder if she also experienced mysterious shooting pains from her groin or if she had sudden "fits" in which she felt "giddy."[10] It would be weird for me to ask—just as it would have been weird for physicians in the late 1800s to ask their patients if they were afraid of gaining weight or "felt fat." On the surface, the absence of information on weight or shape concerns and the presence of lots of physical complaints makes hysterical vomiting seem quite distinct from purging disorder. But it's possible that the core disease is the same, and that these differences reflect the sociohistorical context in which it occurs.

Finally, aside from Dr. Salter's lectures, the treatment outcome of these patients is surprisingly positive. Dr. Salter uniquely conveyed the importance of treatment effectively addressing the neurotic/nervous basis of the disorder and how difficult that could be. In contrast, other doctors described considerable success with very simple interventions. This doesn't match what we see in the treatment of purging disorder, but I also question whether these accounts accurately represent the outcomes for most cases of hysterical vomiting. Publications of the time focused on case studies, with an eye toward sharing what worked. There may have been considerable motivation to demonstrate success. This contrasts with modern approaches of presenting treatment outcomes in samples of many patients, including disclosure of the percentages who did and did not respond to treatment. Further, description of follow-up was limited back then. Some of the patients who recovered so fully and so quickly may not have stayed recovered. A period of temporary remission followed by relapse was demonstrated in Dr. Salter's more complete description of Eliza T. She could be free of symptoms after initiation of a new intervention for up to five days, but then her symptoms would return. This matches descriptions I hear from many with purging disorder. They can stop purging for a while, but then their symptoms return again and again. Perhaps the most that can be taken from treatment outcome in hysterical vomiting is that symptom remission could be achieved through behavioral interventions, supporting that vomiting wasn't linked to infection, food poisoning, or problems with the gallbladder or other parts of the digestive tract.

As tempting as it may be to conclude that hysterical vomiting was purging disorder and to attribute any differences between the two to social context, the DSM-5 already includes a mental disorder characterized by vomiting—it's a somatic symptom disorder with psychogenic vomiting (that is, vomiting caused by psychological instead of physical factors). The modern diagnosis of psychogenic vomiting is defined by *unintentional* vomiting for which no underlying medical cause can be determined and that is unrelated to concerns with weight or shape. Thus, hysterical vomiting may be the historical antecedent to somatic symptom disorder.

During my clinical training, a supervisor gave me an assignment to follow a recent psychiatric inpatient admission for psychogenic vomiting, thinking that my background in eating disorders would make it an interesting case for me. My supervisor was correct—it was an interesting case, but I found my experience in eating disorders to have little relevance or value. My patient, a middle-aged man, explained that he could not keep down water but could drink coffee with sugar. I found myself at a loss to grasp the underlying rules or logic for his condition. Although cognitions around eating can be highly disturbed in purging disorder, there's a common theme related to the effects of eating on weight or shape or sense of control. For instance, I recall one study participant who wouldn't lick an envelope for fear that calories in the adhesive might make her fat. In contrast, my patient with psychogenic vomiting was distraught by how thin and weak he had become and was eager to take in fluids and calories any way he could. He described in great detail the intense stomach cramps that produced uncontrollable vomiting. In purging disorder, the purging is intentional, so it's unclear whether the case reports from the late 19th century would be better considered a somatic symptom disorder or whether they might be historical forerunners to purging disorder. The key would be whether patients experienced their vomiting as intentional or unintentional.

Given that historical accounts from the late 19th century were written when motivations were interpreted as being unconscious, little information or insight is provided into the experiences of the girls themselves. We don't know their explicit motivations or whether they experienced anxiety or indifference toward their vomiting. As a consequence, it's not clear if their vomiting was intentional and probably never will be. In contrast, historical accounts of anorexia provide numerous examples of affected girls and women resisting efforts to make them eat. This may be why Dr. Gull's description of *anorexia nervosa* gained popularity over Dr. Lasègue's *anorexie l'hysterique*—the patients were unmoved by their own starvation. They were unnervingly calm in the face of an illness that was killing them—quite the opposite of how we think of hysteria. We just don't have the same quality of accounts around vomiting in those who weren't underweight from that era or any era before that.

If purging disorder is a new disease or even a modern incarnation of hysterical vomiting, then the features we see today—concerns about weight and shape motivating purging—likely reflect the relatively modern idealization of thinness as a beauty ideal for women. Although it may seem natural that thin is beautiful in our current culture, thin was not always a beauty ideal for women. In the famous painting "The Judgement of Paris" by Peter Paul Rubens (1577–1640), Paris triggers the Trojan War by awarding a golden apple to Venus as the most beautiful among the Roman goddesses, over rivals Juno and Minerva (Figure 2.2). Venus is depicted as a young female with golden hair, fair smooth skin, and rolls of fat around her back, midriff, and thighs with unmistakable dimples of cellulite. This was beautiful not only to Rubens; round, full figures have been venerated for their

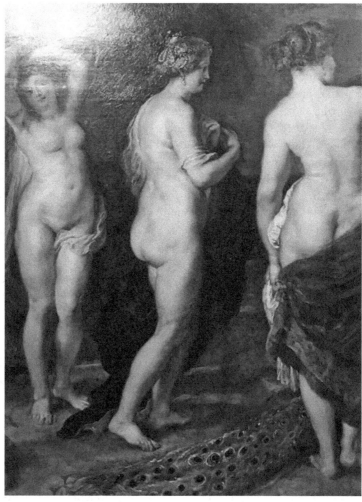

Figure 2.2 Close-up of Aphrodite/Venus as the winner of the golden apple for possessing the greatest beauty in the painting "The Judgement of Paris," demonstrating that ideals of beauty vary across history and cultures.

beauty and value across several cultures—particularly their value in terms of fertility. As we trace images from the Victorian era with their corsets and bustles, a larger posterior was *the* ideal of female beauty long before Kim Kardashian. In times when a fuller figure is the ideal, there may be less pressure to eliminate food through purging, making purging disorder a modern problem in which we have so much available food and so much pressure to keep from getting fat. One approach for tracking whether cultural shifts in beauty ideals contribute to when and where purging disorder emerges is to examine cultures that do not traditionally value thinness as they are exposed to Western media.

PURGING DISORDER IN NON-WESTERN CULTURES

Anthropologist and psychiatrist Dr. Anne Becker has been studying eating disorders in ethnic Fijian girls since 1995. Traditional Fijian culture valued larger female figures as a sign of fertility, acceptance, and love. Family feasts celebrated feeding as an expression of care, and thinness was viewed very negatively because it represented isolation and a lack of family support. In 1995, Dr. Becker was able to ask girls how they felt about their bodies and whether they felt the need to diet to influence their weight. She was also able to give them a survey that asked about bingeing and vomiting. The timing in 1995 was critical because it occurred within one month of when televisions were introduced into the homes of girls' rural villages. In 1995, most girls didn't have a TV in their own homes, and they placed little to no importance on being thin and were generally happy with their bodies. Several endorsed bingeing, but none used vomiting to control weight in 1995. Three years later, however, a new set of 17-year-old Fijian girls expressed beliefs that success, wealth, and independence were related to being thin, and they wanted to be thin. Most had TVs in their own homes and specifically described the influence of shows like *Beverly Hills 90210* on their desire to lose weight. In an interview, one girl shared,

> the actresses and all those girls, especially those European girls, I just like, I just admire them and I want to be like them. I want their body, I want their size. I want myself to be [in] the same position as they are . . . Because Fijians are, most of us Fijians are, many of us, I can say most, we are brought up with those heavy foods, and our bodies are, we are getting fat. And now, we are feeling, we feel that it is bad to have this huge body. We have to have those thin, slim bodies [on TV].[11]

The number dieting to lose weight increased significantly, and more than one in 10 girls reported self-induced vomiting to control weight. In 1998, just three years after TVs were brought into their villages, there were more than two girls vomiting for every one girl who reported bingeing—suggesting that Western television had effectively introduced purging disorder to ethnic Fijian girls between 1995 and 1998. But that's just the first half of this story.

Prior to Westernization, indigenous medicinal herbal purgatives (*dranu*) were used to facilitate feasting in Fiji, consistent with customs that valued a fuller figure as a sign of familial love (Figure 2.3). In 2003, eight years after televisions were brought into their villages, 15% of girls reported vomiting, abusing laxatives, or doing both to control their weight. And 35% described using traditional herbal purgatives, with most purging to influence their weight. For example, one 17-year old girl explained her use: "I was, like, um, very, um, not satisfied with my weight, so I tried Fijian medicine [. . .] I took it and I tried to like make me sick so that I could, uh, vomit and like [. . .] [have] diarrhea."[12] Her body mass index at the time placed her squarely within a healthy weight range—not even remotely overweight—and she was purging weekly. Another 18-year-old girl used *dranu*

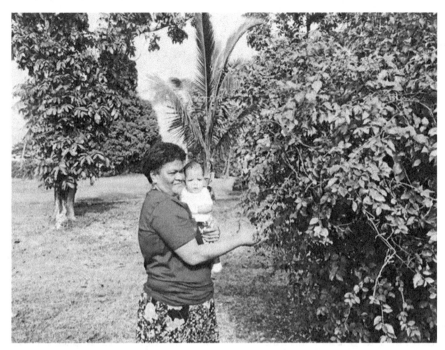

Figure 2.3 A traditional herbal medicine, *Lali* (English translation: "bell"), is used in Fijian culture to help children eat well and cure infections in the tongue and mouth believed to be caused by eating sugary foods. This medication falls into the broader category of *wai ni macake* in Fijian ("medicine for illness characterized by poor appetite and thrush"). In addition, this medication is used to "clean (flush) the stomach" and "reduce belly fat." Strong concentrations cause diarrhea and vomiting and have been used by some Fijian girls to control their weight. Pictured: Sala and Cema. Photographed by Isoa Rokomatu.

to lose weight daily, explaining she used it "just for keeping safe and, uh, control something, control anything that can happen."[13] Most of these girls weren't bingeing. Traditional Fijian practices merged with newly introduced Western ideals to form a culturally specific form of purging disorder that was both more common and more impairing than bulimia.

These patterns are not unique to Fiji. In a study of black adolescents in post-apartheid South Africa, girls ages 14 to 18 years were interviewed in small focus groups drawn from four schools differing in racial composition and wealth. Reflecting both cultural differences in body ideals and varying exposure to Western ideals, girls from poorer backgrounds and predominantly black schools identified emotional stress and physical factors, such as AIDS, tuberculosis, and drug abuse, as primary reasons that some girls get "too thin." In contrast, girls from wealthier schools recognized desires to look thin as a reason to lose weight.

Across all schools, several girls described Zulu traditions of purging to promote health and how their parents gave them laxatives when they were younger. Within their culture, this would be no more alarming or unusual than U.S. parents giving their kids chewable vitamins. Further, girls described how Zulus drink water or coffee to induce vomiting daily to cleanse themselves prior to breakfast. Although all of these represent purging as a behavior, none of these culturally accepted practices is purging disorder. However, these traditions provide a cultural back-drop for the emergence of purging to lose weight and purging disorder after ex-posure to Western ideals of beauty.

For example, girls from all schools acknowledged the use of vomiting and laxatives as a means of weight control by their schoolmates. And one girl from a school located in a historically all-black, low-income urban township admitted that she was breaking from customs by vomiting after she ate breakfast rather than before. In fact, girls from schools with a higher proportion of black and ec-onomically disadvantaged students were more likely to report using traditional Zulu practices to be thin than were girls at the more affluent schools. Yet, most participants didn't think that eating disorders were a problem in the black com-munity, suggesting that purging for weight loss wasn't viewed as an eating dis-order. The authors specifically posited that purging disorder may be particularly common among many black South African females but goes unrecognized be-cause they use culturally sanctioned rituals of purging.[14]

Just as televisions were being introduced to rural Fijian villages, television was introduced to Tanzania in East Africa in 1995. Interviews were conducted in the native language of Kiswahili with girls and women about their exposure to tele-vision, film, internet, and magazines and presence of eating disorder symptoms. Greater exposure to Western media was linked to greater eating pathology, in-cluding the presence of purging disorder in Tanzanian female students—all of whom were at a healthy weight but induced vomiting to control weight in the absence of binge eating.

These ethnographic studies demonstrate the presence of purging disorder in non-Western cultures specifically after exposure to Western media. They also demonstrate how culture shapes the expression of purging disorder. In Western countries, self-induced vomiting is the most common form of purging in purging disorder. In addition, purging disorder is less common than bulimia in the West. In non-Western cultures, we see the adaptation of traditional medicinal practices, such that purging through laxatives and emetics is more common than self-induced vomiting. We also see that purging disorder may be more common than bulimia in non-Western cultures, potentially because its core feature is linked to traditional medicinal practices.

WHAT DO THESE PATTERNS TELL US AND WHY DO THEY MATTER?

Understanding that up to one in five women have suffered from purging disorder at some point in their lives speaks to the public health impact of this illness and to the feasibility of gaining insights through research on how to prevent and treat it. Although all mental disorders are rare, there is a threshold below which it's impractical to invest resources (time, money, effort) to address the problem. If only one person in a country every century had an illness, we could never learn enough about it to help the next person. And, even if we could, it wouldn't make sense given how many people's lives are impacted by other problems for which we don't have solutions. We don't face that barrier for purging disorder. It's common enough that we *can* and have learned a great deal about it. And it's common enough that we *need* to work toward helping those who suffer with it.

Understanding that the disorder is more common in women than in men identifies possible risk factors, both cultural and biological, that may contribute to the disorder. It also points to potential biases in how we define purging disorder. Understanding that the illness develops in adolescence but is not restricted to adolescents, and occurs in all racial and ethnic groups, indicates when prevention should be initiated (before puberty) and may minimize the impact of common biases in who is recognized and helped. As one young man wrote on his own experiences with purging disorder, "I think you are probing a very good subject that is indeed way under-reported and recognized [. . .] Which I want to stress is also a under-reported subsect of that under-reported category, MEN who purge." Finally, observing that purging disorder is relatively modern and watching its emergence in non-Western cultures in response to Western ideals of beauty supports the potent role of cultural factors. Given that purging disorder is defined by the use of vomiting, laxatives, diuretics, or other medicines to influence weight or shape, we have decided that weight and shape must be important factors to the individual. We can see how the importance of these factors varies between genders, over the course of history, and between cultures. Knowing "who, when, and where" gives us insight into why someone develops the illness. But we must remember that the answers to "who, when, and where" also reflect how we define the illness. As we move forward, our understanding of purging disorder must evolve to be inclusive without blurring its boundaries with different illnesses (psychogenic vomiting) or cultural practices that are not even an illness.

Part I of this book addressed four important questions: What is purging disorder? Who suffers from purging disorder? When and where does purging disorder emerge? The answers to these questions lead to the focus of Part II: *Why* does someone develop purging disorder? The answer may seem pretty obvious. A person develops purging disorder because modern, Western culture prescribes an unrealistic ideal of beauty that is too thin for women and too muscular for men. This answer has merit, but it's incomplete. To understand why someone develops purging disorder, we must explore how sociocultural values are transmitted to an individual and the psychological and biological factors that leave some more vulnerable than others to these forces.

PART II

Why Does Purging Disorder Develop?

The Usual and Unusual Suspects

Fear of Fat

This chapter starts with the usual suspects—sociocultural factors—to explain why someone develops purging disorder. I examine cultural beliefs linking weight to health, beauty, character, and popularity and the transmission of these beliefs through media, friends, and family. These sociocultural factors are specific to the development of eating disorders compared to other mental illness. But none of these social factors is specific to the development of purging disorder compared to bulimia. Purging disorder is an eating disorder (vs. a mood or anxiety disorder) because it shares features and risk factors with other eating disorders. Importantly, none of the "usual suspects" completely accounts for why all individuals or even a given individual develops purging disorder. If sociocultural factors could explain all instances, then everyone exposed would develop an eating disorder, and they would all develop the same eating disorder. Only a minority of those exposed to cultural body ideals develop an eating disorder, and even fewer specifically develop purging disorder. In chapter 4, we will explore psychological features that are both shared with other eating disorders and potentially unique to purging disorder to examine why only some people are particularly susceptible to developing purging disorder in response to harmful messages from their social environments. After that, chapter 5 plunges more fully into some "unusual suspects" to describe unique biological factors that distinguish purging disorder from other eating disorders. These factors may explain why someone purges after eating normal amounts of food and does not become underweight.

Fear of fat drives people with purging disorder to engage in extreme methods to rid their bodies of weight. One woman wrote, "I am 5′4 and 118 lbs; [. . .]—I know that purging is not healthy. However, for whatever reason, I feel that if I get to 120 lbs, I feel fat." Another woman shared how following weight loss, "I find myself purging more than I have in the past because I'm afraid of gaining the weight back." These women are not alone. Over 90% of women with purging disorder experience intense fear of gaining weight or becoming fat, and over 90% "feel fat" even though they aren't overweight. Several studies have found that a belief that being thin will make life better, concerns with not being thin enough, and dieting more frequently all predict who develops purging disorder.

A fear of fat and feeling fat trigger anxiety when a person is confronted by fattening food, a distorted reflection from a large window, or an unflattering photo. And people with purging disorder go out of their way to avoid these things. But people must consume food no matter how much they fear its consequences. Purging becomes a means to prevent that food from turning to fat. In some ways, a fear of fat is like a fear of contamination in obsessive-compulsive disorder, and purging is like the compulsive hand washing a person may use to remove dirt and germs.[1] However, there is an important difference between fear of fat and fear of contamination.

Psychological studies support that humans have evolved a predisposition to fear potentially dangerous animals and situations that were deadly to our ancestors. Many people fear snakes, heights, and large bodies of water. Similarly, we possess an inherent revulsion to contamination—whether it's gagging when we smell sewage or vomit or flinching when someone sneezes (flinching reflexively causes us to pull back, hold our breath, and squeeze our eyes shut—a *perfect* response to airborne viruses!). However, in our evolutionary past, people were most likely to die from starvation and diseases that led to wasting. If evolution prepared us to be afraid of anything, it should be a fear of being too thin. Yet, in *Forbes* magazine's most recent list of the 10 highest-paid fashion models,[2] nine were medically underweight![3] This suggests that instead of fearing a leading cause of death in our ancestral history, we celebrate it. Something is overriding what should be an inherent fear of being too thin and driving our fear of fat. Where does a fear of fat come from? It comes from our social environment. But the sources reach far beyond the fashion (or movie) industry, and each source contributes to why a person develops purging disorder.

SOURCES OF SOCIAL INFLUENCE

I often find myself in conversations with people who have never taken a step back to critically evaluate whether being fat is bad. They accept this as a natural truth. Even those who acknowledge how unhealthy most runway models look don't fully grasp how culture has shaped their own feelings about weight. To see how much social factors may have influenced your own thoughts on the topic, I've prepared a brief quiz (Box 3.1). No one else will know your answers, so feel free to answer candidly.

Give yourself a point for every "true" response. The quiz touches on the main messages regarding weight in our society in terms of health, beauty, character, and social acceptance. The higher your score, the more you have absorbed cultural messages about body weight and the more reasons you have to fear fat.

Before getting into the cultural sources of these fears, I want to objectively define fat. Fat is made of networks of carbon, hydrogen, and oxygen that form fatty acids. Fat is found in food and in our bodies. Animal-based foods contain the same fats found in our bodies while plant-based foods contain fats from other combinations of carbon, hydrogen, and oxygen. That's because animals and plants

Box 3.1

BELIEFS ABOUT WEIGHT

1. Being thin is healthy.   T   F

2. Being thin is beautiful.   T   F

3. Being thin demonstrates self-control and strength of character.   T   F

4. Being thin increases your popularity.   T   F

create different sources of energy for their own survival. And that's the thing to remember about fat. Ultimately, it's a source of energy that contributes to survival. Our bodies store fat to support cellular function when food isn't available. Fat helps regulate body temperature to make more efficient use of available food. It permits absorption of vitamins and contributes to the structure of skin, which forms a crucial boundary to protect our bodies against injury and contamination. Scary, right? Or maybe just boring. Fat, in and of itself, is not inherently exciting to most of us (apologies to organic chemists, food scientists, and dietitians). But what I've just described is not what we usually mean when we use the word "fat." Instead we're typically talking about the amount of fat in our food and the amount of fat in our bodies, and too much fat can be frightening. Why? For one thing, we are constantly reminded of the health risks associated with being overweight.

FAT AND HEALTH

According to the Centers for Disease Control and Prevention (CDC), obesity is associated with "the leading causes of death in the U.S. and worldwide, including diabetes, heart disease, stroke, and some types of cancer." [4] The increasing incidence of type 2 diabetes in children has been blamed on increasing rates of childhood obesity, prompting widespread public health campaigns to warn people of the dangers of being overweight. Despite these efforts, body weight has increased steadily and significantly in developed nations around the world over the last several decades, and the majority of U.S. women and men (roughly 7 out of 10 adults) are currently at a weight that falls in the range for being overweight (body mass index [BMI] ≥ 25 kg/m^2) or obese (BMI > 30 kg/^{2}).[5] The average weight for adult women is 168.5 lbs, contributing to a BMI of 29 kg/m^2. The average weight for adult men is 195.7 lbs., also giving a BMI of almost 29 kg/m^2. The problem with the CDC's approach is that it identifies excess weight as the main problem rather than focusing on behaviors.

Composition of food intake and daily activity level are behaviors that influence both weight and disease risk. We use weight as a shortcut to infer whether a person engages in healthy behaviors, but it's just a shortcut. Someone who is overweight can be much healthier than someone whose weight falls within a healthy range. How? A heavier person may eat well-rounded meals, remain physically active, sleep well, and refrain from smoking, drinking and other recreational drug use. This person is taking good care of his or her body. And before rejecting this example as unrealistic because "how could someone be that healthy and still be overweight?" think about the people in your life. How many are carrying "a few extra pounds" while maintaining a healthy lifestyle? Conversely, someone in a healthy weight range may eat an unbalanced diet, remain inactive, sleep poorly, smoke cigarettes, and drink excessively. So, "false" is the best answer to the first question on the quiz because weight, in and of itself, does not indicate health status. Instead, behaviors determine health.

A recent examination of dietary behaviors and death rates in 195 countries found that eating more fruits and eating more whole grains were associated with longer life, again reinforcing the link between healthy behaviors and health.[6] Those behaviors also influence weight, and that's how weight became a shortcut for inferring health. But that doesn't make weight the main problem. It makes it another outcome. Equating lower weight with "healthy" moves us to believe that any means are justified to avoid being fat—even purging. (Chapter 6 delves into the medical consequences of purging to reveal how dangerously misguided this conclusion is.)

What happens if we focus on healthy behaviors instead of weight as a key target for helping people? One truly groundbreaking prevention program did just that. Researchers at the Harvard School of Public Health collaborated with the wellness coordinator for the Boston public schools to develop Planet Health—an innovative school-based curriculum to increase knowledge and specific behavioral changes to form a healthier lifestyle. The program emphasized four changes:

1. Increase daily consumption of fruits and vegetables.
2. Decrease (but not eliminate) daily consumption of high-fat foods.
3. Reduce time spent watching TV or on the computer ("screen time").
4. Increase moderate and vigorous physical activity.

The program used a two-year curriculum for sixth and seventh graders that was integrated into the teaching of four major academic subjects (language arts, math, science, and social studies) as well as physical education. For example, students in math might get a word problem involving nutritional information for packaged food to use fractions in multiplication:

In the checkout at the grocery, you see a king-size package of Reese's Outrageous!™ candy bar, and the nutrition label says that there are 130 calories per serving with 6 grams of total fat, 3.5 grams of saturated fat, and 16 grams of sugar per serving. A single serving is 1/3 of the candy bar. How many grams of fat are in the entire package? (Answer: 18 grams of fat)

This approach ensured that students learned the topic specific to the subject while also learning skills to make healthy choices about food and activity. For recommendations 1 and 2, this might mean buying that king-size Reese's Outrageous!™ bar but sharing it with a friend and making sure that you also picked up an apple or carrots while shopping for snacks.

Ten schools in the Boston public school system were randomly assigned to receive this enhanced curriculum while another 10 used the standard curriculum. Planet Health students increased their fruit and vegetable consumption and reduced television viewing compared with students in the control schools. In intervention schools, girls were significantly less likely to start purging to control weight compared to girls in schools without the program. Planet Health reduced the onset of purging by more than 50% in girls. In addition, Planet Health decreased odds of obesity in girls to half of what was observed in schools using the standard curriculum. Spending less time watching TV predicted decreases in both purging and obesity in girls. These findings support that health is maximized when we focus on health behaviors rather than on weight because improving healthy behaviors reduced purging and obesity risk.

Beyond our culture's unhelpful focus on weight rather than on behavior, our understanding of "healthy weight" doesn't match medical guidelines. According to the World Health Organization, a healthy weight ranges from a BMI of 18.5 to less than 25 kg/m^2. For a U.S. woman of average height (almost but not quite 5-foot-4), this translates into a healthy weight range of 107 to 144 lbs. For a U.S. man of average height (a smidge over 5-foot-9), this translates into a range of 127 to 170 lbs. That's roughly 40 lbs, a large range—much larger than most people realize and much, much larger than experienced by the 5-foot-4 woman with purging disorder who felt fine at 118 lbs but "fat" at 120. While most people don't harbor a two-pound range for what they consider acceptable or healthy, they also don't consider a 40-pound range as healthy. Many of us walk around with a 10-pound range for our "healthy weight."

How did we come to adopt such a narrow range for our idea of healthy weight? Our views of "healthy" weight are skewed by our beauty ideals. We're too ready to accept unrealistic weights as a "healthy goal" because we promote beauty ideals that fall near the bottom and even below the healthy weight range.

FAT AND BEAUTY

Beauty ideals have never matched what women and men generally look like. That's what makes them "ideals." Throughout human history, art has played an important role in reflecting and shaping ideals of beauty and targets of scorn. This remains true today. However, the turn of the 20th century brought about technological advances that merged art and industry with mass production of food and clothes (necessitating the invention of clothing sizes) and mass media, including magazines, movies, television, and, most recently, social media. We are born into media-rich environments that spread ideals of beauty and targets of scorn like wildfire. What's worrisome about current ideals is that they are markedly thinner for women and leaner and more muscular for men than what people really look like. Part of this discrepancy is driven by population-based increases in body weight. Part is driven by an entertainment industry that rejects anything outside of a narrowly defined ideal for women and men. In *Forbes* magazine's most recent list of the top 10 highest-paid actresses worldwide,[7] only one in 10 was overweight or obese. As a group, actresses had an average height of 5-foot-6 and weighed 132 lbs, giving them an average BMI of 22 kg/m^2. If we remove the one overweight actress, on the grounds that her weight is often incorporated into physical humor essential to her comedic career rather than as a defining feature of her beauty, the average weight for top-paid actresses drops to 124 lbs, with a BMI of just under 20 kg/m^2. To reach this ideal, the average U.S. woman would need to lose over 50 lbs (or she could grow 2 inches and then lose 40 pounds). Given the discrepancy (and the options), it becomes less of a mystery why women adopt extreme methods to get or stay thin.

The study of Fijian girls described in chapter 2 provides fairly compelling evidence that media images idealizing thinness contributes to purging. To look at the media's influence in our own culture, we have to look at the same girls over time to see whether purging starts after they absorb cultural ideals of thinness. A study looking at thousands of girls over time found that girls who reported trying harder to look like females on TV, in movies, and in magazines were more likely to start purging at one-year follow-up compared to the girls who weren't concerned with looking like actresses. The researchers continued following girls in this sample for seven years. The same factors emerged—trying to look like women they saw in the media predicted who started purging.

While women today have lived with thin ideals for most if not all of their lives, men's ideals have diverged from reality more recently (at least within my lifetime). For men, fat is bad but thin isn't better. Looking at *Forbes* magazine's list for the top 10 highest-paid actors,[8] we get an average height of 5-foot-11 and weight of 190 lbs, resulting in a BMI of 26.2 kg/m^2. No actor is underweight—not even close: The lowest BMI on the list is 24 kg/m^2. However, this doesn't make them closer to the average BMI of U.S. men because only 1 of the 10 actors is objectively overweight (compared to 7 out of 10 U.S. men). Similar to our actresses, this one exception is a comedian, suggesting that you can be a successful overweight actor or actress if you make people laugh. The other actors have higher BMIs because of their incredible muscle mass. For example, Dwayne "The Rock" Johnson has a BMI over 30 kg/m^2. However, he is not obese. And the men of Marvel (actors portraying Ironman, Captain America, and Thor[9]) are not overweight despite having BMIs above 25 kg/m^2. Adolescent girls and boys are confronted by equally unrealistic ideals, though these ideals for boys motivate excessive weight training, diets that are high in protein and low in fat and carbohydrates, and abuse of steroids—what Dr. Alison Field referred to as a "male version of purging disorder."

There is some good news. Population-based changes in body weight have increased demand for clothing lines that offer larger sizes, and the fashion industry has responded. Since the 1960s and 1970s beauty ideals for women haven't grown any more realistic, but they have grown more diverse and curvy. As we see more changes in who is featured in ad campaigns, our ideals for beauty for women may approach a weight that won't motivate girls and women to purge because they feel fat. The answer to question 2 on the quiz should be "false" because changing ideals for beauty demonstrate their subjectivity—they do not represent factual statements that can be evaluated as "true" or "false." They are opinions, and opinions can change. Unfortunately, for men, changing ideals have grown increasingly unobtainable. But men may be somewhat more protected from another level at which culture influences risk for eating disorders in general and purging disorder in particular. Within Western culture and several Eastern cultures, appearance is a more salient part of women's value than it is for men.

FAT AND CHARACTER

What is the cost of being heavy in a thin-obsessed society? It's substantial because we ascribe all sorts of personal deficits to those who are overweight or fat. Those who are heavy are viewed as weak, lazy, lacking in self-control, and bad. These beliefs begin at an early age. A friend e-mailed me in a slight panic because her son had just started daycare and told her he didn't like his new teacher because the teacher was "fat." My friend was horrified because the teacher wasn't overweight, leaving her to wonder how her three-year-old son had adopted such unrealistic weight ideals and why the teacher's weight would even be a reason to dislike her! I suggested to my friend that her son might not have actually been trying to describe the teacher's bodily dimensions. Instead, he may have been trying to come up with a word that meant "bad"—he was at an age where he knew that fat meant bad but didn't actually understand what "fat" was. With time, children learn what fat looks like and to ascribe all that is undesirable to those who are overweight.

Early in my career I mentored a college senior on her honors thesis, in which she examined children's attitudes towards weight. She created drawings of a boy and a girl at three weights: thin, average, and chubby. She based her study on another project I'll describe shortly. All six illustrations were shown to a sample of girls and boys, ages seven to nine years, and they were asked to rate each child according to eight descriptions: kind, best friend, honest, funny, gets teased, lonely, lazy, and ugly. These ratings were used to create a score for how positively the children rated the figures (with reversed scoring for the last four descriptions). Based on children's ratings, thin was better than average weight, which was better than chubby.[10] However, an interesting pattern emerged depending on whether children were rating pictures of girls or pictures of boys. In ratings of girls, there was a strong preference for the thin girl, with a more modest difference between the average and chubby girl. In contrast, for boys, the preference was roughly equivalent for the thin and average boy, with the worst ratings reserved for the chubby boy. Being overweight was bad for girls and boys, but being thin was only good for girls. This gives boys a wider range of weights associated with positive qualities.

Although being muscular may be a physical ideal for males, quality of character doesn't suffer from failing to achieve this ideal for boys.

In a second college thesis, we looked at attitudes about weight and identity that occurred outside of conscious awareness using the Implicit Association Test (IAT), a measure best known for its ability to detect racial bias at an unconscious level.[11] We revised the measure to detect weight bias and to measure weight identity and self-esteem (Figure 3.1). We recruited men and women with weights that were within a healthy weight range and that fell in the overweight or obese range to complete our modified IAT. Regardless of personal weight, we found weight bias—our participants demonstrated a significant implicit association between "heavy" and "bad." Further, individuals described their weight accurately on questionnaires—supporting accurate explicit awareness of personal weight for both women and men. However, only overweight women demonstrated an implicit association between the "self" and "heavy." Men implicitly paired "self" with "light" regardless of their actual weight. Finally, only women demonstrated an unconscious link between weight identity and self-esteem. At an implicit level, women who identified themselves as heavy also identified themselves as bad.

In chapter 2 I explained that purging disorder was more common in women than in men. Part of this reflects gender differences in idealization of thinness (vs. muscularity), resulting in a larger gap between where women are and what is perceived as healthy, beautiful, and morally good. Another part of this is the extent to which women are more likely to base self-worth on their weight. In interviews of women with purging disorder, they rank weight and shape among the top factors, if not the top factor, influencing how they feel, judge, and evaluate themselves as a person—making it more important than how they do in school or at work, or how they are in their relationships with others, including being a friend, a daughter, or a parent. Men are less likely to prioritize their weight or

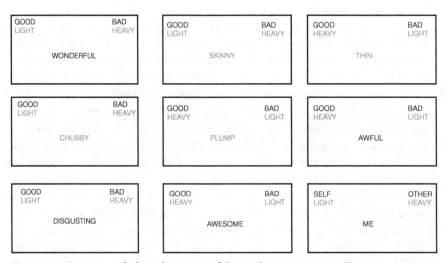

Figure 3.1 Depiction of adapted versions of the Implicit Associations Test to measure implicit weight attitudes and implicit identification of one's own weight.

shape in this way. It might be bad to be fat for a man, but this can be offset by professional success and wealth. This reflects a culture that emphasizes the importance of appearance for women versus performance for men.

Like any form of bias, the association between being fat and being bad is open to confirmation bias. That is, once we accept something is true, we view the world through that lens. Recently, research examined how implicit attitudes toward sexual orientation, race, skin tone, age, disability, and body weight changed from 2007 to 2016. Of these, negative implicit attitudes toward body weight were the only set that has gotten worse.[12] When we think of people who are amazing and thin, we view their bodies as achievements—it's an outward sign of their inner self-control that led to their success. When we think of people who are amazing but not thin, we don't stop to notice that they don't have perfect bodies. Want an example of this? I looked up the last five women and last five men to win the Nobel Peace Prize. A person who works tirelessly and effectively for the good of others demonstrates all of the moral qualities we should aspire to—strength, integrity, courage, caring, intelligence, and generosity. Guess what? None of them looked like movie stars. They came in the full range of sizes, with several of them being significantly overweight. The real people inspiring Oscar-worthy roles look like real people, not like the actors and actresses who portray them. Ultimately, nothing about weight makes a person morally superior or inferior. Going back to that quiz, the answer for question 3 is decidedly "false." Unfortunately, like any form of bias, weight bias becomes a justification for prejudiced behaviors, including weight-based teasing, bullying, and social rejection. This takes us to the fourth reason to fear fat—it's unpopular.

FAT AND POPULARITY

A classic paper published in 1961 established that 10- and 11-year-old children demonstrated consistent bias against obese peers. The researchers created six drawings of a boy and six drawings of a girl. The six versions were matched with one exception—the presence of any physical handicap or limitation. There was a drawing of a boy and of a girl with no physical handicap, ones in which the child had a leg brace and crutches, ones in which the child was in a wheelchair, ones in which the left hand was missing, ones in which the left side of the face was disfigured, and ones in which the child was obese. The researchers then arranged the drawings in a random order in front of a child. Boys were shown drawings of boys, and girls were shown drawings of girls. Without any additional information, the researchers instructed the children, "Look at all these pictures. Tell me which boy (girl) you like best?"[13] After the child responded, that picture was removed, and the researcher asked, "Which boy (girl) do you like next best?" This continued until all pictures had been selected in order from most to least liked, kind of like picking sides for a game in gym class. The researchers did this with 640 children who differed in race and ethnicity, economic background (from poor to wealthy), geographic location (from New York City to rural Montana), and presence of physical handicaps. The children demonstrated an absolutely astounding consistency in their rankings. In every sample and every subgroup, the order I used to describe the six drawings is the rank order for best to least liked, with the obese child coming in dead last. This basic study design and its findings have been repeated and are still true today.

In presenting this study in the classes I teach, I've asked college students to generate explanations for why children produced these rankings. Students have suggested that obese children would be less fun because they couldn't run as fast. But they could run faster than a child in a leg brace or wheelchair. Students have suggested that it's because children want to choose friends who are like them in physical appearance. But several of the children in the study would have been overweight and presumably very, very few would be missing a hand or have a disfigured face. In the end, the reason to reject the obese child extends beyond reasons of physical fitness (health) and physical attractiveness (beauty) to beliefs that weight is under our personal control and that deviating from our cultural ideal is a sign of personal weakness (character). Inferences about the personal failings of the overweight become the justification for all forms of discrimination, including social rejection, and a powerful reason to fear fat.

When the researchers examined the mean rankings of the drawings by girls (of girls) and by boys (of boys), they found that the girls provided even more consistently negative ranks for the disabilities that impacted appearance—specifically, for the child with the disfigured face and for the child who was obese—whereas the boys were somewhat more negative toward the disabilities that impacted physical function (not enough to shift the relative rankings). This means that young girls, who socialize primarily with other girls, face even greater pressure to fear fat. Girls not only judge themselves more on their weight and shape, they can expect to be judged more harshly by their female peers on weight and shape. Although purging may feel shameful, it can be hidden. Being fat cannot. Again, purging may seem like a small concession to make to be accepted.

Remember that study that followed thousands of girls to determine why some of them started purging at one-year follow-up? Girls who reported that being thin was more important to their friends, changing their eating habits when they were with their friends, and dieting more frequently were significantly more likely to start purging than girls who didn't have these experiences.[14] In a separate study of high school girls, those who started purging between fall and spring of their senior year reported that being thin was more important to their friends and that their friends directly modeled disordered eating attitudes and behaviors. My students have shared stories of how the girls in their sororities buy laxatives together and start dieting and purging to achieve beach-ready bodies before spring break. Extending this beyond high school and college, we found that having a college roommate who dieted more frequently doubled the likelihood of using self-induced vomiting to control weight in women at 10-year follow-up, when women were entering their 30s. In this same study, we interviewed women about their experiences in college. Many shared that they had learned to purge from a friend or roommate. They described designated bathrooms in which girls would collectively go to get rid of food they had just consumed in the dining hall. Several reported that when they were in college, it seemed like a harmless behavior—one that they could stop at any time. (In chapter 9 I will reveal how wrong many of them were.)

In interviews of women seeking treatment for their eating disorders, one woman recounted how she was first introduced to the idea of vomiting:

> She remembered her girlfriend's mother describing how some models vomited after eating to control weight. Although the patient initially considered this practice "disgusting," she reported that her first vomiting episode occurred when she weighed herself, considered herself to be over-weight, recalled the conversation with her girlfriend's mother, and decided to "give it a try." From that time on, she engaged in vomiting whenever she weighed herself or judged herself to be overweight. Her vomiting increased when she began college and an older sorority sister explained to her which bathroom was allocated by the sorority for vomiting following parties during which excessive amounts of foods and alcohol were consumed.[15]

In interviews with 24 patients who vomited to control their weight, 10 recalled learning about the practice from friends or acquaintances, and another 7 had read about it.

Is your likelihood of purging related to whether or not someone physically near you is purging? That was the question asked by researchers examining responses from over 15,000 high school students across 144 different schools covering approximately 80 U.S. counties. They found significant clustering of any eating disorder symptom as well as specific behaviors such as dieting, exercising, fasting, and taking diet pills, and some evidence that purging was more likely to occur in clusters. Just like use of alcohol or drugs, teens get initiated into purging as an effort to fit into their peer groups. Data for this study were collected in 1999, before the launch of Facebook or release of the first iPhone. The advent of social media and smartphones has fundamentally altered the nature of social networks and transmission of cultural ideals among peers. Beyond pressure to be accepted by peers in school, young people face pressures to get "likes" from their "friends" and "followers," elevating the association between fat and social rejection to a whole new level.

SOCIAL MEDIA INFLUENCES

Unlike previous generations, today's adolescents and young adults are surrounded by social media. The purging disorder patients I saw early in my career would not have been exposed to social media as a risk factor; back in 2000, Facebook, Instagram, Twitter, YouTube, and Snapchat didn't exist—nor did the smartphones that deliver 24/7 access to updates and images from celebrities, friends and followers. But they exist now, and, with more than 2.5 billion users worldwide, social media outlets actively influence attitudes and behaviors that impact risk for purging and purging disorder.

A few years ago an undergraduate proposed a study for her senior honors thesis examining how using Facebook impacted eating disorder risk. We found that the more time women spent on Facebook, the more disordered their eating. We then invited some of the same women to come into the lab, where they were randomly assigned either to use their own Facebook accounts as they normally would for 20 minutes or to spend 20 minutes reading an online article about the ocelot and watching a brief video on the rainforest mammal. Those who had spent 20 minutes on Facebook reported significant increases in anxiety compared to those who spent 20 minutes learning about the ocelot, and using Facebook reinforced weight and shape concerns, which had actually dropped for those learning about the ocelot. Regardless of what women were doing online, after 20 minutes of screen time, both groups demonstrated a significant decrease in their desire to exercise (inactivity seemed to beget inactivity). The Facebook group felt more anxious, were still concerned about weight and shape, and didn't feel like exercising, whereas the ocelot group felt less anxious, were less concerned about weight and shape, and also didn't feel like exercising. Although using Facebook for 20 minutes didn't cause anyone to start purging (good thing, because it would have been unethical for us to try to induce purging), it created circumstances in which purging is more likely.

Social media use differs from use of traditional media. Not only are users looking at idealized images, they are posting images of themselves—carefully selected and often edited images (Figure 3.2)—to receive likes and comments. One of my current doctoral students, Madeline Wick, examined how editing and posting photos on Instagram impacted eating pathology. Among college students, 1 in 3 women and 1 in 15 men endorsed using smartphone apps to edit their physical appearance before posting photos of themselves on Instagram. Eating disorders were two times more likely in those who posted edited photos compared to those who didn't. Similar to our Facebook study, we then invited some of the students who posted edited photos into the lab for an experiment. After taking participants' photos in the lab, we randomly assigned them to one of four conditions: 1) Edit the photo as they normally would and post it to Instagram, 2) Do not edit the photo and post it to Instagram, 3) Edit the photo and do not post to Instagram, or 4) Do not edit the photo and do not post it to Instagram. We found that posting edited photos caused increased weight and shape concerns. In addition, posting photos, whether or not they were edited, caused increased anxiety and reinforced urges to restrict food and exercise compared to not posting photos. These findings revealed a consistent and direct link between *how* people use social media and eating disorder risk.

These unique qualities of social media could contribute to purging and purging disorder. Before the advent of social media sites, we were confronted with unrealistically thin or muscular images of beauty from magazines, films, and television. We also engaged with peers who represented a full range of expected body weights and shapes in our immediate environment. Now, we have a constant and

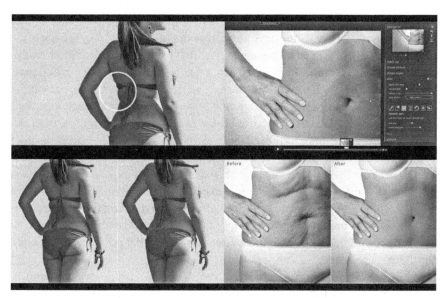

Figure 3.2 Example of tools available to alter photos that promote unrealistic ideals of beauty among peers on social media.

active digital space to engage with peers who may simultaneously portray and reinforce unhealthy body ideals. In addition, posting images of the self to solicit likes is a form of self-objectification. That means treating the self as an object, a thing, instead of a person. Seeking social acceptance based on a passive quality of visual appearance rather than person-based qualities such as kindness, friendship, humor, or intelligence further contributes to undue influence of weight and shape on self-evaluation. In addition, it is much easier to engage in violent acts, such as purging, when the body is reduced to a thing. Finally, you can compare your posts to those of your friends to determine whether you are measuring up. Kristen Bell (celebrity from television, movies, *and* Instagram) coined the phrase "comparison hangover" to capture the consequences of entering this kind of social competition. Given the size of social media circles and bias that goes into what gets posted, you can always find someone who makes you feel worse about yourself. And those same social media apps advertise a range of miraculous products to fix what's wrong. One of my research assistants, a recent college graduate, described how her social media feed was filled with products to eliminate belly fat. Reading through user comments, she discovered that they produced diarrhea. Users see idealized images, post selected images of themselves, often editing what they wish were different about their appearance, which only reinforces that something was wrong with their appearance, and then see ads that make using laxatives seem like a miracle cure for bodily imperfections. In some ways, it's a testament to human resilience that more people don't suffer from an eating disorder.

Peers can transmit broad cultural messages into our immediate social environment to influence risk for purging. But taking a step back, we can see that weight cannot be the sole determinant of social acceptance. Seven out of 10 U.S. adults are overweight, but they aren't all living in complete social isolation. Think of your own friends. Do you only love and care about thin people? Going back to the quiz, weight doesn't dictate whether or not we have friends. In addition, unlike the broader culture into which we're born, we get to choose our friends and partners, and we can choose to change our interactions with them. One prevention program utilized peers to co-lead groups of sorority women to elicit and challenge the thin ideal. Results supported the idea that peers can promote healthier attitudes and behaviors around eating and weight and reduce eating disorder risk. One of my doctoral students, Dr. Tiffany Brown, adapted this intervention to help men with body image concerns and found significant reductions in weight and shape concerns and disordered eating behaviors for men who worked together to reject the lean and muscular ideal. Understanding the powerful impact peers have presents an opportunity to choose friends who support what's best for you and to engage with those friends in a way that prioritizes what's best for them.

While people can choose their friends, people don't get to choose their families. Families and other influential adults provide another avenue for transmitting broad cultural messages into our immediate social environment. Given our cultural beliefs about weight, parents may fear for a child who deviates from weight ideals. And parents' own histories with eating and weight can heighten these fears and their child's risk for purging.

FAMILY INFLUENCES

We live in an era in which eating disorders have become multi-generational problems. A study of thousands of girls followed over seven years showed that having a mother with an eating disorder more than doubled the likelihood that girls started to purge before they reached the age of 14. For high school girls, those coming from families in which relatives engaged in disordered eating and emphasized the importance of thinness were the ones who started to purge—and these effects extend beyond high school. When mothers diet more frequently and fathers make more comments about weight, their daughters experience greater increases in the importance of thinness as they transition from their 20s to their 30s. Among those daughters who became parents over the course of follow-up, that greater importance of thinness increased the likelihood that they worried about their own children's weight—even when they knew that their children were in a healthy weight range. Having a parent describe her 10-year-old child as overweight predicted higher eating, weight, and shape concerns when that child was 14, and this predicted the onset of purging disorder by the time the child reached 17. Finally, from the only twin study of purging disorder conducted to date, we have learned that purging disorder does run in families. Chapter 5 addresses how much of this is explained by genes and how much by family environment, but at least some of it appears to be family environment.

These findings come to life in a troubling story shared by one woman who struggled with purging disorder for over 30 years:

> I remember when I was 14 like most young girls, I had put on about 10 extra pounds and I remember my father stating that he was going to have to call me his little butterball (I only weighed about 118 pounds at the time). I remember I went a whole 7 days without eating anything, not a piece of bread and only drank water. At the end of that seven days, my mother and I were in the car and I told her I had lost a few pounds by not eating all week. Expecting to get chastised, to my surprise, my mother looked at me and said, "keep up the good work, you are looking better." Over the next few years, I found that through purging I would be able to keep my weight down.

CONNECTING THE DOTS

This chapter presents a compelling case for the impact of sociocultural factors on purging and purging disorder. The introduction of TV to Fiji triggered vomiting to control weight in teenage girls. In the United States, girls wanting to look like actresses (which means weighing 50 lbs less than the average U.S. adult woman) were most likely to start purging to control their weight. In a culture where thinness (or muscularity) is a beacon of health, beauty, moral character, and social acceptance, purging seems like a small price to pay to avoid being fat.

Cultural messages are reinforced in our immediate social environment. Some parents model their own concerns with eating and body weight and directly comment to children about their children's weight and eating in ways that increase risk for purging and purging disorder. As children enter adolescence, puberty triggers rapid and dramatic changes in body size, shape, and weight, and peers become increasingly important sources of social values. "Fat talk," often used to reinforce social bonds through sharing vulnerability, can spread feeling fat and fears of weight gain like a virus. Its evil cousins, weight-based teasing and weight-based bullying, use varying levels of coercion to target a person's weight as a basis for social rejection. Linking social acceptance with body weight reverses any biological imperative to avoid starvation with the threat of isolation. Although I think it's possible for someone to develop purging disorder without a specific social influence, this isn't probable. For the vast majority, *multiple* social influences contributed to the illness.

So far, we've followed the story of how we are gaining weight as a population while living in a weight-obsessed culture—pretty much a perfect recipe for any eating disorder, but especially a disorder in which people who are not underweight purge to control their weight. I've also covered how exposure to these ideals through media, peers, and family increases risk for purging and purging disorder. But this isn't a story of gloom and doom. The purpose of identifying risk factors isn't to point fingers at celebrities and "body shame" them for being too thin or too muscular, or for speaking too openly about their own body image, nor to blame friends or parents for the culture in which we live. We have no control over the culture in which we are born, and awareness does not confer immunity. But you can turn that awareness into an intervention to inoculate children from these harmful messages.

Our strongest evidence that sociocultural factors contribute to purging is the success of a program that reduced purging by getting girls to spend less time watching TV. TV viewing both exposes girls to media images that promote the thin ideal, and promotes inactivity that increases risk for weight gain, increasing discrepancy from this ideal. Using the intervention on a school-wide basis, as this program did, also embedded girls in a social environment that promotes healthy behaviors. Peer-led interventions in high school and college-age women and men have reduced internalization of the thin ideal in women and of the muscular ideal in men and reduced risk of developing eating disorders. We may not control the culture into which we are born, but we can actively work together to change messages in our immediate social environment and seek changes at broader cultural levels to reduce purging and purging disorder.

Importantly, even with the most powerful sociocultural interventions, we probably could not completely eliminate purging or purging disorder. In the Planet Health schools, 2.8% of girls started purging to control weight. Social factors alone cannot fully explain why someone purges. As we saw in chapter 2, teenage girls in Fiji purged to look thin but also to feel in control. Cultural messages linking body weight to perceived moral character explain part of why purging would make a person feel in control. However, another part of this stems from how purging influences emotional states. Patients with purging disorder purge unwanted calories *and* unwanted feelings, and the use of purging to regulate emotions suggests another answer to the question "why?" This is explored in the next chapter.

Purging Unwanted Calories
and Feelings

Does risk for purging disorder just depend on circumstances? Is it simply a matter of being unlucky in where (and when) you were born? No, because the vast majority of people never use purging to influence weight or shape. As alarming as it is that over 6% of girls in Boston public schools began purging (that's over 1 in 20 girls!), this also means that 94% of girls didn't. These 94% of girls received the standard curriculum and were exposed to all the cultural messages that instill a fear of fat, but they didn't start purging. This makes sociocultural factors only part of the explanation as to why someone develops purging disorder. To get the rest of the answer we must understand why people react differently to the same circumstances. Simply put, two people can be exposed to the same sociocultural environment and have very different experiences because no two people are exactly alike, not even identical twins raised together (more on this in the next chapter). Two people can sit right next to each other at the same movie and have very different reactions to that movie. Only some people will come out of the latest *Avengers* movie committed to looking like Scarlett Johansson/Black Widow or Chris Evans/Captain America, and even fewer will purge their popcorn. In the last chapter I reviewed evidence that media outlets portray an unusually thin ideal for women—unusual in the sense that most women aren't currently that thin. I also described how girls exposed to these ideals and those who personally aspired to these ideals were more likely to start purging to control weight. This chapter delves into *why* some girls and boys care enough about cultural ideals to start purging.

The differences between us reflect a combination of qualities we're born with and unique experiences we've had growing up. The qualities and experiences linked to differences in how we think, feel, and behave fall into the domain of psychological factors. Not surprisingly, psychological factors are highly relevant to understanding why someone develops any mental disorder, including purging disorder.

Compared to people without an eating disorder, those with purging disorder are more likely to have an anxious temperament and to display greater perfectionism, greater emotional volatility, and a stronger urge to respond to negative feelings with self-harming behaviors. It's not entirely clear how much of this was true before the eating disorder developed, but some of these psychological differences begin very early in life, long before eating disorders appear.

ANXIOUS TEMPERAMENT AND DEVELOPMENT

From the moment of birth, babies differ in how "easy" they are. Some babies eat and sleep well, make cute gurgling sounds with strangers, and are easily calmed and comforted by caregivers. Other babies, not so much. Developmental psychologist Jerome Kagan observed that some babies are consistently shy and fearful from a very early age. These inborn tendencies influenced how these infants responded to their environments—they were more likely to cry in response to strangers. It affected how they acted within their environments—they were more likely to avoid new sounds and new toys. And it affected the responses they elicited from their environments—caregivers were more concerned about protecting their sensitive infants from anything that might upset them. Although temperament is not destiny, it lays the foundation for whether children will be more or less anxious as they encounter new situations, whether they will avoid new situations, and whether others will try to protect them from new situations. An anxious, inhibited temperament sets children on a path to develop a personality marked by negative emotions, a trait called neuroticism. Countless studies support the link between neuroticism (also called negative emotionality) and eating disorders. Indeed, the link is so strong that anorexia and bulimia are officially called "anorexia nervosa" and "bulimia nervosa" in the DSM-5 to denote that these are "nervous conditions" or "neuroses" (this is also to distinguish them from medical terms that specifically mean "loss of appetite" or "excessive appetite," which occur in a range of conditions).

Anxiety is key because it motivates behaviors—it is an inherently activating emotional response. Anxiety increases heart rate, breathing rate, perspiration—all physical responses to support action. But action toward what? In most cases, toward nothing—it's geared for escape, to get away, to avoid. This means that a tendency to experience more anxiety influences behaviors in anticipation of what will be dangerous or upsetting before that upsetting thing happens. This makes new situations particularly daunting because they're unpredictable. Something bad might happen. Apprehension toward new situations is common, and lots of people feel uncomfortable with uncertainty. For those with purging disorder, this uncertainty feels out of control, and purging instills a sense of certainty. As one woman commented, "My best explanation for my purging behavior is that when things felt out of control with some area of my life, I created an artificial crisis in another area that I could then resolve through purging. In that sense, purging was certain validation in an uncertain world." While most people don't love uncertainty, some people absolutely abhor it. The degree of discomfort is related to the expected likelihood that something bad will happen and how upsetting it will be when it happens. For someone high in anxiety, both are elevated. For example, when doing something for the first time, making mistakes is completely normal and receiving corrective feedback is part of the learning process. Those who are very high in anxiety find the prospect of making an error and receiving critical feedback disastrous. To avoid this disastrous outcome, their heightened anxiety motivates an intense focus on detail to get everything right. In her *Purge* memoir, Nicole Johns recalls how her therapist commented that Nicole completed her intake forms with the greatest attention to detail of anyone before her. And Nicole took this as a compliment. This reveals the pathway from anxiety to perfectionism and its pitfalls. The cornerstone of perfectionism is the need to be flawless and pride in striving for this impossible state of being. Numerous studies show that individuals with purging disorder are perfectionists.

PERFECTIONISM: A SOLUTION TO ANXIETY . . . AND A SOURCE OF ANXIETY

In her memoir, Johns describes her perfectionism, how it's been expressed throughout her life, and how it influenced the development and maintenance of her eating disorder. She has a graduate school grade-point average of 4.0. She keeps her room clean and organized. When a vacuum cleaner she uses in the rehabilitation center breaks, she insists she be allowed to use one from another floor rather than leaving her room unvacuumed. Like her, many people with purging disorder have high perfectionism. For many, perfectionism becomes untenable as they hit adolescence.

While it may be possible to achieve a 100% on a seventh-grade math test, how does one achieve a 100% in middle-school friendships? Is it being the most popular girl in the most sought-after friendship circle? Is it always being picked first for basketball and making every shot? No one experiences that. No one can be everyone's favorite person all the time. For someone who is shy, fearful of new situations, and socially anxious, the demands of adolescence are overwhelming. Not only is the body changing in embarrassing and uncomfortable ways, but social demands are growing exponentially, and emotional responses to these changes reach new highs and new lows. It's confusing. In tests of information processing, individuals with purging disorder struggle with a skill referred to as "central coherence"—this is the ability to see the forest for the trees so that you can make sense of a bunch of different little pieces of information. When people are low on this skill, they are more vulnerable to feeling overwhelmed and confused and more likely to experience extreme changes in mood. In one study, researchers found that worse performance on a measure of spatial reasoning predicted earlier age of onset for purging disorder. When you feel confused, you might want to cry out of frustration or for no reason at all, but social norms don't allow these emotional expressions. Adolescents quickly learn to hide their feelings to avoid appearing vulnerable or weak. Middle school in the United States presents a gauntlet of tests of emotional strength through teasing, gossiping, social exclusion, and outright bullying. Those who are more anxious and more perfectionistic are more likely to turn on their own bodies to increase a sense of control.

Focusing one's fears and distress on one concrete outcome—weight or body shape—simplifies the scope of the problem. One woman shared, "I might say that I tend to have to be 'in control,' I can tell if I am 2 lbs overweight. It's interesting, if I am 118 I feel 'perfect.'" Achieving this specific ideal stands for everything a person wants—beauty, strength, popularity, and success—because that's what our culture has taught us from a very early age. It offers a pathway for complete control and eliminates ambiguity and uncertainty. If you can control what you eat, then you can control what you weigh, and this will influence how much people admire you and want to be your friend. Achieving a perfect body is the solution to anxiety over an amorphous array of potential problems. It's also the cause of anxiety because this solution is doomed to fail. We actually have much less control over our weight than we realize (more on this in chapter 5) and being perfect is fundamentally incompatible with being human.

Perfection has a static quality that is poorly suited to survival. To survive as a species, we need variation among people. To survive as an individual, we need variation within ourselves over time. But perfectionism can't tolerate these variations, these differences—the difference between our body and that of an actor portraying a superhero or the difference between the ups and downs within our daily life will always represent distance from an ideal. This makes natural variation a personal failure. Social and personality psychologist E. Tory Higgins identified the gap between self-perception (actual self) and how you think you ideally should be (ideal self) or ought to be (ought self) as key sources of anxiety and depression. Perfectionism ensures that gap by setting impossible standards and increases risk for the later development of eating, mood, and anxiety disorders. In a large sample of women with eating disorders, purging severity was linked to the gap between how women viewed themselves versus how they ought to be.

Putting this together, perfectionism increases the likelihood of feeling bad and decreases tolerance for these bad feelings. Bad feelings such as depression increase purging frequency in adolescents over time, and, combined with dieting and expectations that being thin will solve everything, contribute to the onset of purging disorder. As Johns wrote, "Emotions scare me. Emotions signal a loss of control, and I have tried so hard and for so long to be in control of as many things as possible in my life."[1] Using weight as a concrete objective for intangible strivings is how people who are not overweight come to "feel fat"—it's how the 2-lb difference between 118 and 120 lbs equals the difference between "fine" and "fat." It isn't simply the experience of body size or mass. It's much more than that. "How do you explain to someone—who has never had an eating disorder—that fat is a feeling? To be more precise, fat is a combination of feelings and experiences. [...] By focusing on my body at the precise moment when I am so emotionally uncomfortable, I am deflecting the uncomfortable emotions onto something more tangible—my body."[2] " 'Fat' is code for feeling scared, angry, ashamed, hurt, and sad all in one."[3]

PURGING: A SOLUTION TO DISTRESS . . . AND
A SOURCE OF DISTRESS

At one level, purging is a response to the fear that food will cause weight gain. By getting rid of the food, the threat of fat has been eliminated, at least until it's time to eat again. Yet individuals with purging disorder do not purge all food eaten. Instead, the emotional context of eating predicts what food is kept down and what food is expelled. When a woman feels angry and desperate, vomiting to the point of exhaustion alleviates her distress and gives her a temporary sense of control. "Instead of feeling my anger, I throw it up."[4]

One of my doctoral students, Dr. Alissa Haedt-Matt, undertook a detailed study of emotions surrounding vomiting in women with purging disorder. To do this, she asked women to carry small handheld computers[5] with them so that they could record their current feelings as they went about their daily lives. Women responded to six random signals from the computer throughout the day for two full weeks. In addition to responding to these random signals, women completed ratings after purging to capture when they purged and how they felt after vomiting. Over the two weeks, women provided 1,978 momentary ratings of mood in response to random signals and another 154 ratings after purging. Clear patterns emerged when we compared mood on days with purging to days without purging. Greater sadness, anxiety, anger, and shame characterized the days that women purged.

Clear patterns also emerged for how mood changed before and after purging (Figure 4.1). In the hours leading up to purging, women had high negative emotions that only got worse as the day progressed without any increase in positive emotions. In the hours after purging, women experienced a significant decrease in negative emotions, suggesting that purging had "worked" to alleviate their distress. In addition, on days that purging didn't occur, positive emotions— feeling happy, calm, relaxed—increased over the course of the day. Many studies

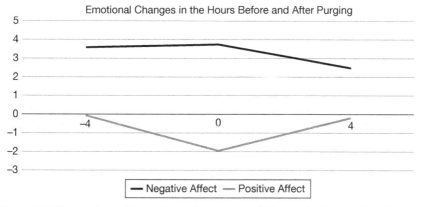

Figure 4.1 Changes in positive and negative emotions before and after purging relative to changes observed over days without purging in women with purging disorder.

have examined emotions leading up to and then following purging in eating disorders. Across studies and samples, distressing emotions increase in the hours and minutes before a purge and then decrease after purging. The experience of purging followed by a decrease in distress results in people learning to use purging to control their feelings. This is classic operant learning through negative reinforcement originally defined by behavioral psychologist B. F. Skinner.

By fusing emotions with a feeling of fatness, purging provides an efficient solution. After purging, patients feel control over what is in their bodies. They have pushed back the threat of weight gain and pushed back the negative emotions that spurred purging. Instead of an emotional explosion, the body spews out its vile contents, creating a moment of dissociation—a moment of calm distance from feelings—a sense of control. Purging controls a wide array of problems—weight, emotional distress, physical discomfort—giving it a cathartic, cleansing, controlling allure that people return to again and again. It doesn't matter that purging is ineffective at weight control.[6] It matters that it's effective at emotional control—at least in the short term.

Given that purging reduces distressing emotions, why do people need to keep on purging? If it works so well, why doesn't it make itself obsolete? Because it works well for a little while, long enough to be reinforcing, but it doesn't address the original source of distress. Whatever contributed to increased anger, anxiety, shame, or guilt before purging, it probably wasn't the fact that the person felt disappointed in themselves for not having purged enough that day. It was something else, and purging doesn't tackle the original source of distress—an argument with a friend, negative feedback on an assignment, or a never-ending to-do list. As one woman wrote, "It seems to come and go in intensity depending upon the stress in my life. Right now, I am struggling with the purging disorder again and I'm getting scared because it is ruining my teeth and my stomach feels bad most of the time. I can't stand this and I'm weary." With no effective means to address or adapt to stressors, the stressors come back again and again, like waves crashing onto the shore, eroding the person further, leaving them more vulnerable to purging.

In addition to providing an ineffective long-term solution to emotional distress, purging has its own negative emotional consequences. Although overall distress goes down after purging, one study found that purging predicted increased distress as well as additional purging throughout the evening. How can this be? How can distress both go down and go up after purging? Anecdotally, women tell us that the effects of purging vary by specific emotion. The activating emotions, anger and anxiety, go down. Purging drains the fuel for these feelings. Exhaustion is incompatible with anger and anxiety, but it's not incompatible with sadness, loneliness, or shame. Working with Cara, I came to understand that all of these "calmer" negative feelings curl up inside the void left by purging and plant the seed of worthlessness that makes the impact of stressors so much harder to endure. In the moment, purging creates a sense of control. After that moment passes, it leaves a profound sense of fragility.

Giving up purging means accepting bad feelings and waiting for them to go away on their own time or using adaptive coping to address stressors (more on this in chapter 8). This is how most people cope with feeling bad, but most people don't experience as intense a need for control combined with such an intense range of emotions—that's part of the mental illness in purging disorder. It's not just anger, it's rage. It's not just fear, it's terror. It's not just sadness, it's desolation. And even as someone is feeling these intense, painful emotions, they feel guilt and shame for having such intense, painful emotions. They feel personally responsible for failing to be happy. And this shame deepens the commitment to dampen those feelings and make them go away. Just as reducing vague and intangible sources of distress into "feeling fat" makes it seem manageable, taking physical action on those distressing feelings creates a physical release. As one woman put it, she had developed "an addiction to release." But, for some, purging is not enough.

PURGING AND SELF-HARM

Cara was disgusted by the idea of being fat. She also reported deep-seated hatred toward herself and a desire to kill herself. The first six months of our treatment focused on expanding her reasons to live. Sessions ended with me extracting a promise that we would see each other next week and that she'd call me if she felt she couldn't keep herself safe. Slowly, over the months, we were able to move beyond reasons to live and discuss reasons to live well—that is, the reasons to stop hurting herself with purging and harsh self-criticism over imaginary flaws. We talked about activities she enjoyed (biking, spending time with friends, listening to music) and how to spend more time on activities that made her happy and made her feel strong. The frequency of her purging decreased, and she looked healthier and sounded stronger and happier. She was even able to use humor to challenge some of her deeply held beliefs about her personal value and its association to her weight. I was relieved that we weren't talking about whether or not she would kill herself but also worried that she was still purging. Clearly, we weren't done, but we were in a relatively stable place. That is, I thought we were—until I left the country for two weeks for my honeymoon. I prepared Cara for my absence about two months in advance, arranged for a therapist who specialized in eating disorders to be available to Cara, and reminded her of the resources available to support her safety while I was gone.

When I returned, Cara described how the prior weeks had gone for her. Her purging increased and spread to foods that were normally safe. She had taken a knife and scrawled the word "hate" into her stomach. She got drunk and started a fight with a much larger male acquaintance who "beat the shit out" out of her. Up until this point, I was worried by how little I seemed to be helping Cara stop purging. After this point, I realized that our work together had been allowing her to contain her urges to hurt herself to purging. I recognized that she came to our sessions every week—never canceled, never no-showed. Cara was amazing in her dedication to working on getting better—even when the purging persisted long past the time I told her it would get better. Later in the course of our treatment, after she moved to another town, she took a train for more than an hour each way to keep our weekly sessions. All of this reinforced to me how deeply ingrained the problem was and how easily it threatened to expand beyond the traditional confines of an eating disorder.

Like Cara, people who purge enlist an array of harmful behaviors to escape negative feelings. They are more likely to cut, burn, and bruise their skin, abuse alcohol and drugs, attempt suicide, and die by suicide than those who don't purge. In each instance, we see a reckless disregard for the integrity of the physical self. Where others naturally fear and avoid painful experiences, those with purging disorder seem relatively unaffected. It's as if in exchange for their intense emotional experiences, they actually have blunted experiences of physical pain. Really, it's a tradeoff. People with purging disorder exchange feelings of anger and anxiety for feelings of shame and defeat. They exchange feelings of nausea, bloating, and stomachache for aching throats, raw knuckles, and sore anuses. But it did not start out that way for them. In a journal entry from December 2001, Johns had written, "I made myself sick and it felt really good. I liked it." An April 2004 journal entry reads, "I feel like I'm dying."

What would make someone engage in potentially harmful acts to escape emotional distress? According to clinical psychologists Stephen Whiteside and Donald Lynam, a specific facet of impulsive personality they called *negative urgency* explains this tendency. A large study of adolescents found that higher negative urgency combined with the belief that being thin will solve life's problems predicted which girls developed purging. People do not start purging to hurt themselves, but after repeatedly hurting themselves through purging and other means, they teach themselves that they are worthy of abuse. It's like an abusive relationship with oneself. There are promises to stop and get better that are broken again and again, until the person with purging disorder stops believing their own promises. One concerned husband shared that his wife's purging was linked to her anxiety and poor body image and that "It's so bad at times that she has even scratched her skin because she gets mad at herself because she feels fat and ugly. [. . .] no matter how many times I tell her how beautiful she is or how good she looks in an outfit it doesn't even seem to make a difference." He also asked if her purging might be related to her history of child abuse. He added, "It's actually dawning on me that as a child she had no control over what adults did to her and now this is her way of controlling something in her life." Across eating disorders, those who purge are more likely to have a history of childhood trauma, including physical and sexual abuse.

Taken as a group, individuals with purging disorder are more likely to engage in harmful behaviors toward the self when they are distressed compared to those without eating disorders. But they are not a homogenous group. Even among those with purging disorder, there are differences in negative urgency. These differences translate into the severity of illness and presence of related mood, anxiety, and substance use disorders. Self-destructive behaviors cluster together— people who use multiple purging methods (for example, using both self-induced vomiting and laxatives) are more likely to attempt suicide, drink excessively, use drugs, and report histories of trauma. On the other end of this spectrum, there are high-functioning individuals with purging disorder who report being well adjusted, with childhood histories unmarred by emotional or physical abuse. Weight and shape may be at or near the top of their list of things that influence their self-evaluation, but they place great importance on their relationships with others and with their educational and occupational endeavors. They still suffer from their perfectionism, but they aren't crippled by either emotional dysregulation or an overcontrolled, rigid personality. This range within purging disorder reflects the range within eating disorders and is one reason that people underestimate the severity of eating disorders.

You could easily meet two people with purging disorder who are very different from one another. Yet both would probably challenge the idea that purging is a problem for them, for very different reasons. For one, the purging may seem like the least of their problems. In the midst of substance abuse, self-harm, and suicide attempts, the use of vomiting and laxatives to control weight would not rise to the top of the list of urgent problems that need to be addressed. For the other person, purging may seem like a minor problem for someone who is otherwise doing very well. Yes, she vomits weekly when she feels that she's had just a bit too much—perhaps a dessert she didn't really need—but otherwise she's doing well at work and at home, and has healthy relationships. No one would ever guess she was purging, and is it really more worrisome than other bad habits like smoking or occasionally drinking too much? This kind of thinking leads to an underestimation of the severity of purging disorder and of all eating disorders. Look at Cara. To the outside world, she looked fine. She was college educated, working full time, and had meaningful relationships. She also hated her body at such a profound level that she was able to engage in acts of violence against herself and to seriously contemplate suicide. Chapters 6 and 9 will each examine the consequences of purging and purging disorder to challenge facile assumptions that purging isn't a serious problem.

PSYCHOLOGICAL FACTORS CONTRIBUTING TO PURGING AND PURGING DISORDER

Purging disorder develops during adolescence, particularly during that transition from late adolescence to young adulthood. Being born with an anxious temperament makes the challenges of adolescence more daunting. Combine this with a cognitive style in which it's hard to see the forest for the trees and this time can be overwhelming. Perfectionism represents an effort to control threats by being flawless, and our culture provides a convenient focus for perfectionist tendencies: body weight. Our weight is supposed to be completely under our control, ensuring our health, beauty, moral strength, and popularity. An anxious temperament also increases the likelihood of experiencing emotional distress, and perfectionism widens the gap between how we view ourselves and how we "should" be, which further nurtures feelings of anxiety and depression. Perfectionism also tells us that being unhappy is our fault and that emotions should be controlled. Experiencing emotional distress as a form of bodily discomfort—as "feeling fat"—moves people to view purging as a solution rather than a problem. This is amplified if that emotional distress is also experienced as feeling bloated, nauseated, and having a stomachache—emptying the stomach becomes a logical response. It reminds me of the nursery rhyme, "There was an old woman who swallowed a fly." We don't know why she swallowed the fly, but she swallowed a spider to catch the fly and then continued consuming ever-larger animals to kill the prior animal until "she swallowed a horse." The simple rhyme teaches us how responding to a problem with a short-term solution can generate new problems. Purging begins as a short-term solution to a problem, but quickly becomes a problem itself.

Chapter 5 explores biological factors that influence temperament as well as those that impact body weight and eating. Ultimately, purging disorder is a disorder of eating, and eating is regulated by numerous biological factors that have evolved to support our survival. Indeed, a key step in moving from an anxious temperament and perfectionism to a disorder characterized by purging (instead of or in addition to something else, like obsessive-compulsive disorder, body dysmorphic disorder, or social anxiety disorder) may result from a person's biological makeup. Differences in our biological makeup, starting with our genes, provide another answer for why someone develops purging disorder.

5

Feeling Sick

Genetic and Neurobiological Contributions

So far, I've described why someone develops purging disorder from sociocultural and psychological perspectives. Culture creates values around body weight that our immediate social environments can reinforce or buffer us against, and those values guide how we cope with psychological distress. For those who adopt a "lose weight and everything will be fine" strategy, purging brings temporary relief from distress. A learned association between purging and relief maintains purging as a response to distress even when purging brings on its own problems. Although that explanation is true for purging disorder, it isn't specific to purging disorder. It's the same explanation we would give for binge eating in bulimia or fasting in anorexia. My own research focuses on the complex interplay of biological responses to food intake to explain why someone develops purging disorder versus bulimia versus no disorder at all. This chapter describes my findings and results from other studies seeking to identify biological factors that contribute to the development of purging disorder.

Given the strength of evidence for cultural and psychosocial factors, why would I even look at biological factors? The answer is quite simple—eating is crucial to our survival. That means it's influenced by numerous biological factors. Even though the case for cultural and psychosocial factors is compelling, it's not complete.

Some bodily functions necessary for survival do not require conscious thought or active decisions. For example, we breathe and our hearts beat outside of our conscious control. Some bodily functions required for survival do not require conscious thought but can be controlled or delayed when appropriate. For example, our bodies filter impurities from our blood to produce urine without any planning on our part, but we do control when we urinate—within certain reasonable limits. If a person pushes the bladder's capacity too far, then urination occurs. Some bodily functions required for survival require conscious thought and active decisions but are still strongly influenced by biological drives and regulators. Eating falls into this last category, along with drinking fluids, sleep, and other processes that we can't live without but can choose how we accomplish.

Because everyone has experience with eating I'm not going to focus here on the conscious processes that go into food choices—like what and where to eat. Instead I will glide past a large body of research in that area to zero in on what our bodies do *outside* of our conscious awareness to make sure that we eat enough food to survive. The other reason I will not delve into this research is that none of it has been conducted on individuals with purging disorder. As we get further into this chapter, it will become clear why it's unwise to expect results from neuroimaging studies of bulimia to reflect what's going on in purging disorder. We'll start with evidence from large studies focusing on biological factors that predict purging disorder onset.

In a study of pregnant women and their children, the Avon Longitudinal Study of Parents and Children (ALSPAC), researchers followed the children over an extended period of time to determine factors that predicted the onset of eating disorders, specifically examining factors linked to anorexia, bulimia, binge-eating disorder, and purging disorder. Compared to children who remained healthy, girls and boys who later developed purging disorder had a somewhat lower BMI earlier in life (between ages two and six years). However, after the age of five to six years, their BMI started increasing so that they were heavier than children who remained healthy. Similar patterns were observed for bulimia and binge-eating disorder, except that girls who went on to develop bulimia started exhibiting higher body weight by two years of age. In contrast, girls and boys who went on to develop anorexia had lower BMIs as toddlers and continued to have lower BMIs leading up to when they developed their eating disorder. Given that none of these children had an eating disorder at two years of age and most were free of eating disorders at six years of age, this suggests that biological factors may have been driving differences in their eating behaviors and weight in directions consistent with the eating problems that form the central features of various eating disorders. It also may explain why those with purging disorder are more fearful of fat and gaining weight and why they aren't underweight after they resort to purging. Although body weight is a biological variable, similar to blood pressure, it can be influenced by children's social environments. Thus, another explanation for these early differences in BMI might be related to children's family environments. This raises the question of what factors influence body weight—and do they also influence eating and eating disorders?

GENETIC VERSUS ENVIRONMENTAL CONTRIBUTIONS

Although we tend to think of our genes as providing a blueprint that we carry with us throughout our lives, the influence of genes can change over our lifespans. One of the most obvious examples comes from the effect of sex chromosomes (XX vs. XY) on physical development. From birth, boys and girls differ from each other physically, but many more differences emerge during puberty—and these differences are linked to the influence of hormones in activating additional genetically based differences. So, what do developmental changes in genetic effects mean for BMI? Researchers tried to answer this question by studying a sample of 87,782 twin pairs from around the world (that's 175,564 people) for whom BMI had been measured starting in childhood and through adolescence. They found that the contribution of genes to BMI increased with age. Prior to the age of nine, 40% to 60% of BMI was related to genetic makeup, 20% to 40% was related to rearing environment, and about 20% was related to everything else (officially, these are referred to as "**Additive genetic**," "**Common environment**" or "shared environment," and "nonshared **Environment**," respectively, and abbreviated as "ACE"). But beginning around age nine, genetic factors explained about 75% of BMI, and rearing environment dropped to the point of contributing nothing to BMI by the age of 19.

Going back to that study of BMI trajectories prior to the onset of purging disorder or other eating disorders, this means that genes probably contributed to about 50% of BMI and children's rearing environments explained another 30%. However, by the time children had developed their eating disorders, their BMI was largely explained by their genes. What about their eating disorders? One concerned mother reached out to me to share that she had purging disorder but also to ask "whether or not it is hereditary, because I see the signs in my 10-year-old daughter." Another mother wrote of her experiences as a "practicing purger" when she was in her 20s because she thought she had found "the perfect diet," but now her daughter, currently in her 20s, purges. How much of purging disorder is explained by genetics?

A number of other twin studies from around the world have been used to better understand eating disorders. One twin study has examined purging disorder, and a handful of others have focused on self-induced vomiting or compensatory behaviors more broadly. What have these studies told us? First, across eating disorders, genes contribute to self-induced vomiting. Specifically, in answering the question "why does someone use self-induced vomiting to control their weight?" at least part of the answer can be found in their genes. Indeed, across studies of adult twins, genes explained over 50% of someone's risk for developing recurrent self-induced vomiting. The rest is due to everything else—with no contribution from rearing environment.

Which genes might code for vomiting risk? It's not clear. Although no single gene causes purging, there's probably something in our genes that makes it possible for us to vomit—otherwise, we wouldn't be able to. There is precedent for this in nature: For example, rats are incapable of vomiting. So in addition to having genes that permit us to walk on two legs, talk, and lack tails, we also have genes that make it possible for us to vomit. But we don't know which genes they are, and we don't know which variants might produce someone who is more likely to vomit versus someone who has an iron stomach. I personally know individuals on both ends of this continuum—specifically, my children. One of my sons has a very sensitive gag reflex. If he coughed too hard as an infant he would start vomiting. He also has a more sensitive stomach in general and has been more likely to miss school because of vomiting, and to experience vomiting as a side effect of certain medications. My other son has been sick with vomiting precisely twice in his entire life.

In addition to contemplating the existence of genes that contribute to vomiting ability or vomiting liability, it's worth considering genes that lay the foundations for our temperaments. Remember that shy, fearful, inhibited infant? As much as 60% of temperament comes from genes. So, how much does this explain the heritability of purging? One twin study examined how compensatory behaviors, including purging, were linked to personality, including both negative emotionality (related to neuroticism) and constraint (related to impulsivity). Consistent with everything covered in the previous chapter, higher negative emotionality and lower constraint (i.e., higher impulsivity) were associated with greater use of compensatory behaviors. Similar to results from other twin studies, genes contributed to more than 50% of risk for compensatory behaviors, and genes explained over 30% of someone's level of negative emotionality and over 50% of their constraint. Finally, all of the association between use of compensatory behaviors and these personality traits was explained by genetic factors. Thus, the genes that contribute to neuroticism and impulsivity are the reason that these personality traits contribute to later development of compensatory behaviors. This provides a very different perspective on the link between temperament and disordered eating, suggesting that genes that contribute to anxiety and sadness also contribute to using compensatory behaviors. This could mean that compensatory behaviors are a culturally influenced impulsive response to distress and that the selection of this *specific* coping response to distress is related to genes that increase risk for vomiting, distress, and impulsivity. However, this study also identified genetic contributions to compensatory behaviors unrelated to personality. In fact, over 90% of genetic contributions to compensatory behaviors came from something other than the genes that gave rise to these personality traits.

Importantly, these studies examined compensatory behaviors or self-induced vomiting across all eating disorders and included very few cases of purging disorder. One large twin sample from Australia had a greater number of twins who were purging without binge eating (3.3% of over 1,000 twins). In this study, genetic factors explained only 8% of risk for purging. Most of the risk was explained by nonshared environment—that "everything else" factor.

The only twin study to focus specifically on purging disorder also found that nonshared environment explained the lion's share of risk. Although some combination of genetics and rearing environment contributed to the development of purging disorder, accounting for 44% of risk combined, it wasn't possible to determine how much of that was related to genes versus how much of it was related to the rearing environment. Results may change as new twin studies on purging disorder are published, but these initial findings suggest that genetic makeup is relevant to the development of purging disorder, but that genes may be slightly less relevant for purging disorder than for anorexia, bulimia, or BED (Figure 5.1).

The relative contributions of rearing environment and genetic makeup reflect the roles of sociocultural environment and biological factors, but what does nonshared environment represent? In talking with a student about findings in eating disorders, she asked me whether all biological factors were genetic. They're not. Although all genetic factors are biological, not all biological factors are genetic—some are environmental, like exposure to a flu virus. And this means that some environmental effects are social, and some environmental effects are

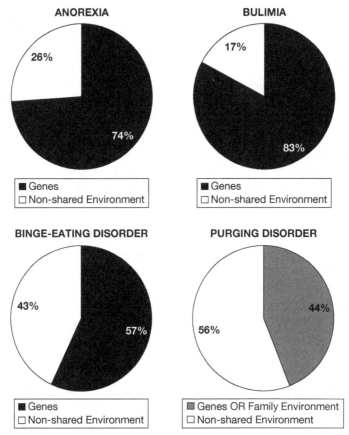

Figure 5.1 Highest estimates for contribution of genes versus shared family environment and nonshared environment to risk for developing eating disorders.

biological. Within a twin study where twins have been raised together, nonshared environment is anything that makes one twin different from another. Using the term "environment" makes it sound like a social factor—something in our interactions with others, and that is one possible example. This could be a specific social interaction, a bad relationship, or a traumatic event that happens in the life of one twin but not the other. But this could also be a biological factor, such as one twin taking birth control pills and not the other. Sometimes, it's both. Specifically, a traumatic event can trigger a biological change in the body that influences the expression of genes. This is referred to as an *epigenetic effect*.

EPIGENETIC EFFECTS

In that large study of pregnant women and their children, ALSPAC, the researchers examined the mothers' reports of how well they felt cared for during their childhoods and then collected samples of the mothers' DNA. This study examined two genes for oxytocin (the so-called love hormone) because oxytocin is involved in forming emotional attachments in relationships. They then looked at the genetic code for these two genes, quality of care, and their interaction to see if this could explain differences in the women's own history of eating disorders. Those with purging disorder reported low care from their mothers when they were growing up compared to women without eating disorders, but there were no differences in oxytocin genes. Conversely, those with bulimia or restrictive eating disorders had a different genotype for one oxytocin gene compared to those without eating disorders, and those with bulimia were more likely to have the combination low maternal care and a specific type of the other oxytocin gene. This last finding suggests an epigenetic effect. Carrying the risky gene code for one of the oxytocin genes was associated with having bulimia only when women also had experienced poor maternal care. Otherwise, carrying that gene type was benign. Similarly, poor maternal care alone was not enough to produce bulimia in the absence of the risky gene. Conversely, for women with purging disorder, poor maternal care alone (rearing environment) was associated with their eating disorder regardless of their oxytocin gene type.

In a third study from the large sample of pregnant women and their children, researchers identified which women had a history of an eating disorder, had an eating disorder during their pregnancy, or never had an eating disorder. When their babies were born, the researchers sampled blood from the babies' umbilical cord. They used the blood samples to determine the extent to which the infants' DNA (the molecules that make up their genes) had a chemical (a methyl group) attached to the DNA or were free of this chemical. Prior research had shown that pregnant women with lower body weights had babies with less of this chemical attached to their DNA (referred to as *demethylation*), and that demethylation predicted lower body fat during infant development. The chemical in question tends to reduce expression of genes—that is, it tends to muffle the effects of genetics on outward traits. Thus, demethylation contributes to a more robust expression of genetic influence, including genetic risk. The researchers found that mothers' eating disorder history predicted demethylation of their babies' DNA. Demethylation was most pronounced in babies of women who had an eating disorder during their pregnancy compared to babies of women with a past eating disorder history, who in turn had greater demethylation compared to babies born to women who never had an eating disorder. When they broke the women down into those who had histories of different kinds of eating problems, they found that the effects were strongest in those with a history of dietary restriction and those with a history of purging without binge eating. In chapter 3, I reviewed how having a mother with an eating disorder more than doubled the likelihood that girls would start purging before they were 14 years old. There we focused on how parents might increase risk by directly modeling the importance of thinness, but some of this environmental effect could influence biological risk for purging disorder too.

Recall my earlier discussion of how the impact of genes on BMI changes over development. This is another example of an epigenetic effect. When children are younger, their parents have more influence over their eating, and rearing environment will have a more direct impact on eating behaviors and BMI. This reflects the influence of environment on genetic expression of traits. Also, as girls move through puberty, they experience a surge in ovarian hormones and cyclical changes in hormones with the onset of menstruation. These hormones create a biological environment that alters the expression of genes and may explain why risk for purging disorder increases during adolescence. Specifically, genes contribute to over 50% of risk for compensatory behaviors (and other eating disorder features) in 17-year-old twins, 14-year-old twins, and 11-year-old twins who have entered puberty. In contrast, genes contribute to 0% of risk for such behaviors in 11-year-old twins who haven't started puberty. That suggests that puberty triggers activation of genes that not only contribute to development (growth spurts, getting one's period, hair in new places) but also to risk for developing specific eating disorder symptoms. And this effect is specific to girls. Boys show no change in heritability of disordered eating over pubertal development. For girls, the ovaries produce hormones that trigger pubertal changes, and there's evidence that these hormones are responsible for the pubertal change in genetic risk for eating disorders.

Why? Let's think about the conditions under which many women are more likely to vomit when they are not actually sick—like the first trimester of pregnancy. Pregnancy represents another time when ovarian hormones increase dramatically, and for some women this causes morning sickness and vomiting. It's possible that the same biological processes triggered by pregnancy hormones are triggered by pubertal changes in hormones to make some girls more vulnerable to vomiting in response to feeling they've eaten too much, feeling upset, or feeling out of control. When women are pregnant, they understand these feelings represent morning sickness, but when girls are going through puberty, these feelings may make them feel like they've eaten too much, especially if they are already concerned about their weight. Different responses to pubertal increases in hormones could be expressed as physical sensations of bloating, nausea, and stomachache that increase risk for purging after eating normal amounts of food.

If purging disorder has a biological cause that does not depend on culture to trigger it, we'd expect to see examples of the illness outside of its current sociohistorical context, potentially in the same demographic group. Returning to those cases of hysterical vomiting from the late 1800s, we see that hysterical vomiting predominantly affected the same subgroup of the population— adolescent and young adult females. Here is another striking similarity between hysterical vomiting and purging disorder: patients with both describe intense stomach pain, bloating, and nausea and an overwhelming urge to vomit after consuming normal amounts of food.

Are there biological differences in those with purging disorder that might contribute to these experiences? My own research has sought to answer that question. My findings support that biological responses to food intake trigger the sensations of nausea, stomach pain, and urge to vomit experienced by women with purging disorder.

BIOLOGICAL CORRELATES OF PURGING DISORDER

To explain biological correlates of purging disorder, I need to describe a little bit about how the food we eat triggers sensations of fullness not just in our stomachs but also in our brains. As a species, humans are diurnal creatures—we tend to sleep at night when it's dark and be awake during the day. This means we eat during the day, and hormones help synchronize the activity in parts of our brain involved in eating to help maintain a schedule of regular eating and sleeping. One of these hormones is called *ghrelin*—the so-called hunger hormone. Ghrelin is released from the stomach, is absorbed into the bloodstream, crosses the blood–brain barrier, and plays an important role in triggering sensations of hunger by activating parts of the brain that stimulate eating and suppressing parts of the brain that terminate eating. When we fall asleep at night, ghrelin levels are at their lowest—giving us a reprieve from hunger that allows us to relax and get to sleep. While we sleep, our ghrelin levels remain low but gradually build while we sleep and peak when we wake up in the morning. So right before you feel ready to eat in the morning, a hormone that triggers feelings of hunger is at its highest level. As you eat, nutrients from food enter your stomach, and those nutrients suppress the stomach's release of ghrelin, causing ghrelin levels to drop dramatically. With the drop in ghrelin, you experience a drop in hunger because the parts of your brain that were driving eating become less active, and the parts that terminate eating become more active. But ghrelin is only one of several hormones that impact eating.

As we eat, the food we consume travels through our stomach into our intestinal tract, where cells release hormones that affect how full we feel. Some are released within 10 to 30 minutes of eating and function as stop signals. Cholecystokinin (CCK) and glucagon-like peptide 1 (GLP-1) are released from the intestines and absorbed into our bloodstream shortly after we start eating, with levels peaking around 15 to 20 minutes after eating. Unlike ghrelin, they don't cross the blood–brain barrier to directly impact brain function. Instead, they stimulate the activity of a nerve that travels from the stomach directly to the brain, known as the vagus nerve. This long, powerful superhighway of information directly stimulates parts of the brain near its base, where the brain meets the spinal cord. This stimulation triggers a signal to those same parts of the brain that regulate food intake. However, CCK and GLP-1 increase activity in the parts that stop food intake and decrease activity in the parts that drive food intake. Have you ever noticed that after you start eating, even when you know that you've probably eaten enough, it can still take a while to feel satisfied? The time it takes for food to travel through the stomach to the intestines, trigger release of gut hormones, and for those hormones to trigger the vagus nerve to activate the brain explains the delay in feeling satiated.

Finally, some hormones, like peptide tyrosine tyrosine (PYY) are also released from the intestines in response to food intake, but PYY levels rise over the course of two hours after we eat. Like ghrelin, PYY crosses the blood–brain barrier to directly impact brain activity. Unlike ghrelin, PYY stimulates activity of brain areas that stop food intake and decreases activity in areas that drive food intake. In addition to directly impacting brain function, PYY stimulates the vagus nerve, that superhighway to the brain, to also suppress food intake. Unlike CCK or GLP-1, PYY levels change gradually and over an extended period of time. Rather than providing the short-term signal to stop eating that terminates a meal, PYY provides an extended signal after the end of a meal to delay when you start the next meal. If you've ever found that your afternoon snack ruined your appetite for dinner, you have PYY to thank. In fact, you have both ghrelin and PYY to thank for the fact that you were so hungry for the afternoon snack in the first place. Towards the end of the two-hour period after lunch, PYY levels were falling just as ghrelin levels were beginning to rise. Taken together, approximately two hours after your last meal, your CCK, GLP-1, and PYY levels are all low, and your ghrelin levels are high again (although not as high as they were when you first woke up) (Figure 5.2).

Figure 5.2 illustrates how the various hormone levels change over the course of a day in relation to food intake when everything is working the way it's supposed to. But how do these hormones function in people with eating disorders? My initial interest in purging disorder grew from my concerns that it might not meaningfully differ from bulimia. I wanted to know if biological disruptions found in patients with bulimia would also be present in those with purging disorder. Specifically, women with bulimia had been found to have a blunted CCK response to food intake compared to healthy women. Several studies had shown that when you gave both groups the exact same food to consume and measured their hormone levels before and after eating, women with bulimia released less

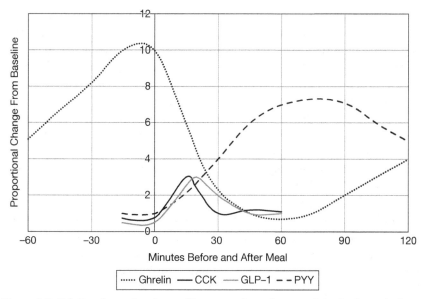

Figure 5.2 Relative change in release of hormones from the gastrointestinal tract before and after food intake that influence food intake.

CCK. It was as if their bodies had been given less food! Given the role that CCK plays in telling the body to stop eating, this could explain the large binge episodes in bulimia. It would be much harder to stop eating once you started if your body wasn't registering how much food you had eaten. But what about purging disorder? To answer this question, we recruited three groups of women: women with purging disorder, women with bulimia, and women without eating disorders. We specifically recruited women with bulimia who purged so that the only difference between women with bulimia and women with purging disorder was the amount of food eaten before purging.

When we interview women in our studies, we ask them to describe in detail a time when they feel that they've eaten too much. And then we ask if they felt a loss of control over their eating during that episode. For healthy women, they report amounts of food that may be larger, but not unusually large. We mostly hear about dinners at restaurants with large portions or picnics or holidays. Importantly, our healthy participants don't experience a loss of control over their eating, and while they may feel like they ate more than they usually eat, it isn't more than most would eat in that context. For women with bulimia, they report amounts of food that are much larger than what most people would eat. Across our studies, women reported consuming approximately 3,000 calories in a single episode, and they experienced a loss of control over their eating. Specifically, they felt like they couldn't stop eating once they had started, often eating until everything was gone. In a *New York Times* article about her experiences with binge eating, Jane Brody wrote, "I would spend the night eating nonstop, first something sweet, then something salty, then back to sweet, and so on. A half-gallon of ice cream was only the beginning. I was capable of consuming 3,000 calories at a sitting. Many mornings I awakened to find partly chewed food still in my mouth."[1] In contrast, women with purging disorder reported amounts of food that do not exceed what most people would eat—about 600 calories on average across our studies—but they experienced this as a loss of control. In Box 5.1 I've given examples of how eating differs when those with bulimia versus those with purging disorder feel a loss of control over their eating. When individuals with bulimia binge, they tend to eat foods they normally avoid, foods high in calories, in addition to eating larger quantities of food. When individuals with purging disorder feel a loss of control over their eating, they often violate their dietary rules but don't consume an excessive amount of food (though it still feels like too much food for them).

In addition to interviewing women about their eating, we brought women into the lab so that we could measure how much food they ate to feel "full." We gave women a standardized breakfast to eat in the morning and had them come to the lab in the afternoon. In a private room, they completed ratings of how they felt right at that moment, consumed frozen yogurt until they felt full, and then completed ratings on how they felt right after eating. All participants were served a quart of frozen yogurt and asked to eat until they felt full. Our participants took less than 15 minutes to reach that point, and all three groups reached the same level of "fullness" based on self-report. However, women with bulimia ate significantly more than healthy women or women with purging disorder to reach

Box 5.1

How eating differs when those with bulimia versus those with purging disorder feel a loss of control over their eating

Loss of Control Eating in Bulimia	Loss of Control Eating in Purging Disorder
• Subway 6-inch Spicy Italian sub—double meat, provolone, banana peppers, black olives, red onions, oil, vinegar, pepperoni, ultimate cheesy garlic bread (1,170 cal) • 1 pack Doritos Nacho Cheese (250 cal) • 2 double chocolate cookies (420 cal) • 2 peanut butter cookies (440 cal) • 1 pint Ben & Jerry's Chocolate Fudge Brownie ice cream (1,040 cal)	• Subway 6-inch turkey sub—turkey, lettuce, tomato, green peppers, cucumbers, pickles, wheat bread, no cheese/no sauce (250 cal) • 1 pack SunChips Harvest Cheddar (210 cal) • 1 double chocolate cookie (210 cal)
Total: 3,320 cal	Total: 670 cal

the same level of fullness, and we found no differences between healthy women and those with purging disorder. Women with bulimia consumed almost 2.5 cups (or almost 5 servings) to feel full whereas the other groups consumed less than 1.75 cups (less than 3.5 servings), meaning that women with bulimia required about 40% more food to feel the same level of "fullness." Importantly, we did not ask women to binge or lose control or "let themselves go." We just wanted to see how much food it took for their brains to get the stop signal from their bodies. Although there were no differences in feelings of fullness after the meal, the groups differed in feelings of nausea, stomachache, and urge to vomit. Healthy women experienced very low levels of any of these before or after the meal. In contrast, both women with bulimia and women with purging disorder experienced significant increases in all three after eating—even though the women with purging disorder hadn't eaten any more than the healthy women had eaten. Both healthy women and women with purging disorder ate less than a pint of frozen yogurt, but only women with purging disorder felt sick afterwards and wanted to throw up.

Based on their own reports and what we observed in the lab, women with purging disorder stopped eating before they ate a large amount of food. Given this, we wanted to know how their bodies physically responded to food intake. To answer this, we needed to have the three groups of women consume the exact same amount of food so that we could measure how their hormone levels changed in response to food intake. If women with bulimia have a lower CCK response to food intake and this is specifically linked to their large binge episodes, would women with purging disorder have a greater CCK response? The answer is yes. Compared to women with bulimia, women with purging disorder had a significantly greater CCK response to food. Women with purging disorder looked very similar to healthy women in CCK function. These findings provided the first evidence that women with purging disorder differ from women with bulimia on an objective biological response. Without this finding, there was a nagging concern that the only difference between purging disorder and bulimia might be a difference in what women were willing to tell us about their eating. However, the differences in observed food intake in the lab and the difference in CCK response supported that women with purging disorder had a different pattern of eating compared to women with bulimia. More importantly, the observed differences in CCK might explain differences in their symptoms.

When we looked at GLP-1 function, we found the same general pattern. Again, women with bulimia had lower GLP-1 levels compared to women with purging disorder and healthy women despite having eaten the same amount of food. And, again, women with purging disorder did not differ from healthy women. Overall, it looked like we had found one reason that women with purging disorder didn't eat more than healthy women to feel full and why both groups ate significantly less food to feel full compared to women with bulimia. Their fullness signals were intact.

When we looked at ghrelin, we found a different pattern. Compared to healthy women, both women with bulimia and those with purging disorder demonstrated higher fasting (pre-meal) ghrelin levels. Although ghrelin levels decreased after eating in all women, the levels remained higher in both eating disorder groups. Yet changes in subjectively reported hunger did not remain higher in both eating disorder groups. For women with bulimia, hunger stayed higher after eating compared to reports from healthy women and women with purging disorder. Furthermore, just like we saw when women ate to the point of feeling full, women with purging disorder reported significantly greater increases in nausea and stomachache after eating compared to both the women with bulimia and the healthy women, even though they all ate the exact same amount of food. What was going on? The answer was that longer-term hormone response to food intake.

Approximately 30 minutes after eating, when the major changes in CCK and GLP-1 are done and ghrelin is low, PYY levels start their climb. However, for women with purging disorder, the PYY level was climbing much more rapidly and going much higher than it was in women with bulimia or healthy women. Imagine that as you were eating, your body was giving you all of the normal signals of fullness and maybe even slightly higher signals of hunger that you felt you had to resist to prevent weight gain, but then *after* you ate, *after* you had committed to whatever you were going to eat, your body responded as if you had eaten a *much larger* amount of food than you had actually eaten. That's effectively how the bodies of women with purging disorder were reacting, and those dramatic increases in PYY contributed to their increased nausea, stomachache, *and* urge to vomit.

These biological responses to food and the reports we get from participants in our studies map on to what women with purging disorder report feeling after they eat. In describing the nausea she experienced, one woman in her mid-twenties explained, "It is hard because I will sit at home and have a tomato for a snack, and that one little tomato will make me run to the bathroom and get it back out. The feeling when I'm done is of great relief." In asking about his daughter, one father wrote, "she doesn't really binge, she claims her stomach often hurts after she eats and the purging makes it feel better." One husband shared that his wife purged because "she gets full real fast even when eating small meals." One man wrote, "From my personal experience, it is the feeling of a bloated stomach that shamed me into purging." In this last experience, we see how the physical sensations of eating and fullness contribute to emotional distress for those with purging disorder, strengthening the relief purging provides.

REASONS PURGING DISORDER DEVELOPS

This is the last chapter focusing on why someone develops purging disorder. If you have purging disorder and you're like the countless people who have contacted me or the numerous women who have volunteered for our research studies over the years, you will recognize some of these answers as being true for you. But I understand that there is a gap between the explanations I've presented and your experiences. Part of this is because there is no one reason that someone develops purging disorder. In considering how important eating is to survival, we're looking at a system that is protected by numerous cultural, social, cognitive, emotional, and biological processes. An eating disorder develops after disruption at multiple levels. Despite exposure to the same cultural messages about weight and eating, most people don't develop purging disorder. Despite experiencing the emotional turmoil of puberty and adolescence, most people don't develop purging disorder. Even among genetically identical twins who are reared together, we see pairs in which one has purging disorder and her twin does not. Something happened to the twin with purging disorder that triggered her eating disorder that didn't happen to her sister. This means that there are multiple reasons that someone develops purging disorder, and the relative impact of each factor will differ across individuals.

One answer might be the differences we see in biological responses to food intake. However, it might not be true. Some biological factors distinguishing women with purging disorder might be consequences of the illness. Repeated vomiting after eating might leave the body unused to food passing from the stomach into the intestines. This could increase the body's sensitivity to any food that makes it through, and increased sensitivity could cause excessive biological responses to that food. This is conjecture. No one has shown that this is true. And it's clearly not true in those who binge and purge. But we do know repeated purging changes many bodily systems. This knowledge broadens our perspective from asking what causes purging disorder to looking at what also happens after purging disorder develops.

A key challenge for interpreting biological differences in women with purging disorder is that eating affects biological functions, and any disorder of eating will disrupt biological functions. This is one reason this chapter appears right before the chapter on medical consequences of purging disorder—some of the biological differences we find in purging disorder might actually belong in the chapter on medical complications of purging. The food we take into our bodies serves as the fuel for brain activity and the building blocks for the hormones we measure. Thus, any alteration to eating could alter the very factors we're examining as possible causes of the disorder. And yet these changes could still be important in understanding illness maintenance. Even if elevated PYY response is a consequence of purging, an exaggerated PYY response could trap individuals into a vicious cycle in which normal amounts of food make them feel sick. This adds to our understanding of why someone develops a disorder characterized by recurrent purging.

Imagine a person born with a genetic predisposition to higher body weight, higher negative affect, and a more sensitive stomach. Imagine this person born into a culture that idealizes thinness—equating it with health, beauty, moral strength, and social acceptance. Imagine this person born in a family that particularly embraces these social values so that they are exposed to dieting and the use of disordered eating as solutions rather than problems. Imagine this person entering puberty, and if this person is a girl, experiencing a surge in hormones that activate changes in her body and her emotions as she's trying to gain acceptance among her peers by being perfectly in control. Her higher BMI is a threat to her social acceptance, and perfectionistic strivings combined with a thinking style that prefers simple concrete solutions make her weight seem like the easiest problem to fix. But dieting isn't enough—particularly when she's out with friends and trying to fit in by eating what they eat. Maybe she hears about purging online or through a friend or even a relative, and one time when she's particularly upset with herself and what she's eaten, she gives it a try. She experiences immediate relief and a sense of control over herself. The next time she feels upset or fat or both, she purges again. Over time, her body may react to purging by becoming more sensitive to the food she does eat so that normal amounts of food trigger excessive satiety responses. Now, she doesn't just feel upset and fat after eating, she also feels physically sick to her stomach. The only relief comes from purging, but purging no longer seems like a simple solution because it brings shame and isolation. But what are her alternatives? She's still not very thin. If she stops purging, she'll just gain weight, and her culture and upbringing have left her terrified of being fat.

Chapters 3, 4, and 5 cover a range of reasons that someone might develop purging disorder. Many of the risk factors are shared with why someone develops any eating disorder. But some of these factors appear to be unique to purging disorder, and these differences are highly relevant when developing treatments for someone with purging disorder. Returning to a question posed in Chapter 1, do we need another eating disorder? We do if we want to capture differences in biological function that might contribute to better treatments.

PART III

Help! Why and How to Get It

6

Medical Consequences of Purging

When my son was starting second grade, he got very sick. We took him to the pediatrician because he was extremely pale and reported that his heart "felt funny." After running initial lab tests, the pediatrician told us that he needed to be admitted to the hospital to have more tests run. The staff were offering him toys to keep and were especially friendly considering it was after 5 p.m. on a Friday. So I asked what they were testing him for, and they responded that his symptoms and bloodwork were most consistent with leukemia. And I responded, "I'm sorry. This may seem like a weird question, but what is leukemia again?" I know what leukemia is, but my reaction was to look for an alternate definition of the word *leukemia* rather than accept that my seven-year-old child might have cancer. I could not comprehend that something so serious could be happening to my child, and being offered medical terminology rather than a more familiar label, such as bone marrow cancer, was a barrier. He didn't have leukemia, but the episode underscores the importance of *understanding* what is wrong—no matter how scary.

My approach in this chapter is to explain medical consequences in layman's terms. Formal medical terms appear in italics in parentheses following everyday language so that I can introduce important phrases without them getting in the way of comprehension. In addition, the medical terms and their everyday definitions appear at the end of the chapter in alphabetical order. That way, if you have a question for a physician, you can refer to the list to get meaningful answers. You can also use this list to search for more information to stay abreast of new findings that will come out after this book is published. If the terms get in the way, just slide past the italicized words in parentheses and don't worry about the list at the end of the chapter.

In chapter 1 I described the different methods of purging: self-induced vomiting, misuse of laxatives, misuse of diuretics, and misuse of other medications. Although all purging methods forcefully evacuate matter from the body, they differ in how they produce their effects. Some medical complications, like severe loss of bodily fluids (*dehydration*), occur across all methods of purging because water is the key matter being evacuated from the body. Importantly, this means that anyone who purges from a fear of fat should understand that, for the most part, they're not ridding their body of fat. They're mostly ridding their body of water. Other complications are specific to the type of purging. About two-thirds of those with purging disorder use one purging method, and self-induced vomiting is the most common.

COMPLICATIONS FROM SELF-INDUCED VOMITING

Individuals with purging disorder often gag themselves by touching the back of the throat (*pharynx*) to induce vomiting. Gagging causes the stomach to clench, and rhythmic stomach contractions push food back up to the mouth through the passage that carries food from the throat to the stomach (*esophagus*). Vomiting also pushes fluids and stomach acid up through the esophagus, throat, and mouth. The loss of fluids causes dehydration. Dehydration places an incredible strain on the body to perform its normal functions because water is essential to support the structure and function of everything in our bodies.

Dehydration can cause low blood pressure (*hypotension*) and impacts heart rate, specifically causing a rapid (*tachycardia*), slow (*bradycardia*), or irregular heartbeat (*cardiac arrythmia*). The decreased volume of water in blood increases stress on the kidneys to filter blood. Dehydration can lead to kidney failure, coma, and death. Indeed, if you found yourself stranded on a desert island, securing drinkable water would be your first priority to increase your chances of survival.

In addition to expelling fluid, vomiting brings stomach acid up through the esophagus, throat, and mouth—all places it's not supposed to be. In the stomach, acid breaks down food for digestion. Cells lining the stomach release chemicals that neutralize acid, and a protective coating of mucus prevents acid from burning through the stomach. That protective coating doesn't extend to the throat or mouth. When stomach acid reaches the throat (*laryngopharyngeal reflux*) or mouth, it eats away at bodily tissue just like it would digest a piece of steak. This causes a burning in the throat and irritates the vocal cords, contributing to hoarseness. In response, the throat may coat the vocal box (*larynx*) with thick mucus, the tissue may thicken, and small blood vessels may expand (*telangiectasia*), making it difficult to speak.

When stomach acid reaches the mouth, it causes ulcers and bleeding. Stomach acid can kill tissue that produces saliva (*necrotizing sialometaplasia*), which along with dehydration contributes to dry mouth (*xerostomia*). Stomach acid also erodes tooth enamel, weakening teeth and contributing to cavities (*dental caries*). The biting surface (*occlusal surface*) of teeth at the back of the mouth and the inside surface (*palatal surface*) of front teeth experience the most erosion. The longer a person vomits, the more likely they are to lose enamel on the inside and outside surfaces of teeth by their cheeks (*buccal surfaces*). One mother expressed concern because her daughter's teeth were showing damage from vomiting three to five times per day. Another woman described how "the enamel on my teeth is getting thin due to the acid." Another shared, "I'm getting scared because it is ruining my teeth." And another simply stated, "I've lost a lot of teeth." Once the enamel is lost, stomach acid erodes the layer below the enamel (*dentin*), which increases the risk of tooth death. Patients who vomit experience tooth pain and receding and inflamed gums (*gingival recession* and *gingivitis*). Both dry mouth and cavities contribute to bad breath (*halitosis*). Many patients brush their teeth after vomiting to rid their mouths of the sour aftermath of their purge. However, brushing teeth and gums weakened by acid increases tooth and gum erosion.

Vomiting causes swelling of the glands located between the mouth and ear that produce saliva (a condition referred to as *parotid sialadenosis* or *sialomegaly*). In addition to altering appearance, the swelling can be painful. Swelling of the parotid glands gets worse in the days following the end of a period of intense vomiting. This can lead some patients to experience themselves as having a "fat face" and redouble their efforts to restrict and vomit.

High vomiting frequency shifts the acidity of blood, which triggers the kidneys to eliminate potassium from the bloodstream. The dehydration caused by vomiting can also trigger the kidneys to eliminate sodium. In addition, stomach fluid contains potassium chloride and sodium chloride. Thus, vomiting causes loss of salts from the body through altering kidney function and through expelling it from the body. Both potassium (K^+ in a periodic table) and sodium (Na^+) are positively charged atoms (*electrolytes*) that are critically important to how cells function throughout the body. Low blood concentrations of potassium (*hypokalemia*) and sodium (*hyponatremia*) shift the balance of electrolytes. When I shared this with Cara to explain why I wanted her to see a physician for a medical workup, she explained that she had read about this and drank a lot of Gatorade after she purged. While I appreciated her ingenuity, I reinforced that a physician would be in a better position to determine whether she needed supplements, to make sure she got the right supplements, and to make sure that any supplements were working with follow-up bloodwork.

Hypokalemia can result from self-induced vomiting, laxative misuse, or diuretic misuse and is particularly likely when a combination of purging methods is used. Hypokalemia is an important medical complication because potassium impacts heart and kidney function. Nerve signals throughout the body are transmitted electrically by shifts in charged particles (also known as ions or electrolytes). Electrolyte imbalances strain the heart and the kidneys and contribute to irregular heartbeat, heart attack (*cardiac arrest*), and kidney failure (*renal failure*). Electrolyte imbalances can also trigger electrical surges in the brain (*seizures*) and cause muscle weakness and muscle twitches. Severe hypokalemia and dehydration from multiple purging methods has been linked to the breakdown of muscle tissue (*rhabdomyolysis*). The clinical symptoms of rhabdomyolysis include muscle weakness, tender muscles, and dark, tea-colored urine. This is a medical emergency that requires inpatient treatment. The condition is typically treated with hydration through intravenous fluids but may require dialysis in cases of severe kidney damage.

During gagging with a finger, the back of the hand scrapes against the upper teeth, causing calluses on the hand, known as "Russell's sign," named for the physician who first described them among patients with bulimia (Figure 6.1). In the

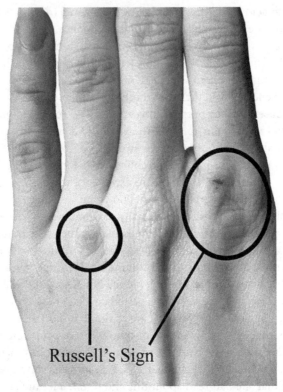

Russell's Sign

Figure 6.1 Calluses on the back of the hand from repeated scraping of knuckles against upper teeth during gagging to induce vomiting, also known as "Russell's sign"—named after Gerald Russell, the physician who first named bulimia nervosa in the medical literature.

1980s, "gag me with a spoon" became a pop-culture phrase to convey disgust by referencing the use of a spoon to induce vomiting. Poking the back of the throat with any object can rip the lining of the throat and cause bleeding. This risk increases when the throat is already raw from repeated acid exposure.

The physical effort of vomiting, heaving while bent over a toilet, bursts the small blood vessels (*capillaries*) in the eyes and on the face, leaving red smears of blood on the surface of eyes (*subconjunctival hemorrhages*) and small red spots on the face (*facial petechial hemorrhages*). Widening of small blood vessels makes them appear like red threads or spiderwebs on the skin's surface. Patients have also experienced reddening around their mouths (*perioral erythema*) and a rash of purple spots on their face that fade with time (*temporary facial purpura*). During vomiting, particles of vomit may be accidentally inhaled, leading to lung infection (*pneumonia*). Pneumonia symptoms include a cough that doesn't subside, fever, shortness of breath, and chest pain. Prompt treatment is imperative to prevent the infection from worsening. Forceful vomiting can break the small, horseshoe-shaped bone that anchors the tongue (*hyoid bone fracture*), which is painful and can make it difficult to swallow or speak. The force of vomiting increases pressure and strain in the abdomen. This can cause rare but serious problems including pushing the upper part of the stomach through the large muscle separating the abdomen and chest (*hiatal hernia*), bursting the main blood vessel that takes blood from the heart to the stomach (*gastric artery rupture*), and tearing tissue surrounding the stomach. Vomiting has been linked to torn tissue connecting the stomach to the spleen (*gastrosplenic ligament*), tears in the membrane anchoring the stomach to the abdominal wall (*greater omentum*), and rips in the base of the esophagus where it meets the stomach (*Mallory-Weiss tears*). In very rare cases, forceful vomiting has caused the stomach to slide up and get folded into the esophagus (*gastroesophageal intussusception*) and pushed the rectum out the anus (*rectal prolapse*). One woman shared that her purging left her with a ruptured intestine requiring three weeks of hospitalization, which she credited with curing her purging disorder.

Repeated vomiting weakens a contracting muscle ring (*lower esophageal sphincter*) that separates the esophagus from the stomach. This makes vomiting easier over time, and many patients describe vomiting as being "automatic" or uncontrollable. One mother wrote that her daughter vomited even when she didn't want to because, according to her daughter, "it just comes up and I can't stop it." The weakened muscle ring allows stomach contents to bubble up unexpectedly into the esophagus (*gastroesophageal reflux*), where the acid causes heartburn (*retrosternal burning*). Although years of antacid commercials have made heartburn seem like no big deal, it can feel like intense chest pain that people confuse with a heart attack. Cancer in the esophagus has been linked to repeated vomiting in both a case study of a 31-year-old woman (*squamous cell carcinoma*) and medical record reviews of eating disorder patients. Importantly, other behaviors often linked to vomiting, such as alcohol and tobacco use, may further increase risk.

Once upon a time, pharmacies sold Ipecac Fluidextract and Ipecac Tincture for home use to induce vomiting if a child accidentally ingested something poisonous. However, these forms of ipecac were removed from the shelves of U.S. pharmacies due to substantial medical risks of misuse—including accelerated heart rate (*tachycardia*), low blood pressure, damage to the heart muscles, congestive heart failure, and death. Ipecac Syrup remains available in a 1-fluid-ounce bottle for the purpose of poison control. However, this does not make it safe.

COMPLICATIONS FROM LAXATIVE AND ENEMA MISUSE

Laxatives and enemas increase elimination of solid waste (bowel movements, stool, poop). Different kinds of laxatives produce their effects by triggering different physical changes in the body. Laxatives can increase bowel movements by increasing nondigestible fiber in the intestinal tract (bulking agents), causing the stool to absorb more water (stool softeners or emollient laxatives), stimulating contractions of the intestinal wall (stimulant laxatives and prokinetic laxatives), changing electrolyte balance in the intestines to increase water in the intestinal tract (hyperosmotic laxatives and saline laxatives), and/or reduce absorption of water by the intestines to increase water in the intestinal tract (lubricant laxatives). When the active agent (for example, sodium phosphate in a saline laxative) is injected into the rectum, it is referred to as an enema. As a group, enemas involve injecting liquid (or sometimes gas) into the rectum to flush solid waste from the bowels. Some of the medical consequences of laxative misuse depend on the kind of laxative used. Similarly, some of the medical complications of enema use depend on what is injected.

Many laxatives are available over the counter, making them easy to obtain and abuse. Stimulant laxatives, such as bisacodyl or sennosides, are fast acting, typically working within 6 to 12 hours, and are therefore particularly prone to abuse. Stimulant laxatives containing phenolphthalein used to be common in over-the-counter medications but have been banned by the U.S. Food and Drug Administration (FDA) due to medical risks; however, they continue to be available in other countries. Phenolphthalein increases the risk of some cancers and causes softening of the bones (*osteomalacia*). Softening of the bones leads to abnormal bone formation and pain at night and when weight is put on the bone, and increases the likelihood of fractures. Stimulant laxatives, containing aloe, cascara, frangula, and rheum, increase the risk of colon and rectal cancer (*colorectal cancer*). The abuse of senna, another stimulant laxative, has been associated with acute liver (*hepatic*) failure. A severe problem linked to the use of stimulant laxatives more than three times per week over a year is damage to the muscle nerves of the colon (*loss of haustral folds*), which contributes to bloating, a feeling of fullness, abdominal pain, and inability to completely empty the bowels (a collection of signs and symptoms referred to as a *cathartic colon*).

The FDA also released a safety warning about the use of over-the-counter sodium phosphate laxatives and enemas. Taking more than the recommended dose has been linked to kidney damage, heart problems, and even death. These risks are elevated in those experiencing dehydration. Additional complications linked to enema use come from bacterial infections from using nonsterile equipment or injecting contaminated liquids, burns from injecting liquids that are too hot, and damage to or even perforation of the bowel. The National Center for Complementary and Integrative Health within the National Institutes of Health noted that "Colon cleansing procedures may have side effects, some of which can be serious" and that "'Detoxification' programs may include laxatives, which can cause diarrhea severe enough to lead to dehydration and electrolyte imbalances."[1]

Other laxatives are only available by prescription. Prokinetic laxatives, such as metoclopramide, found in the prescription medicine Reglan, have been used for the treatment of irritable bowel syndrome and work within 30 to 60 minutes of an oral dose. However, many prescription prokinetic medications have been removed from the market by the FDA or have "black box" warnings due to serious potential side effects. FDA regulations and warnings only impact medications in the United States. While the medical consequences of misusing prescription laxatives tend to be greater than for over-the-counter formulations, this does not make over-the-counter laxatives or even fiber supplements harmless.

Bulking agents, such as psyllium or methylcellulose, take approximately 12 to 24 hours to take effect. However, depending on the source of nonsoluble fiber and the amount consumed, some fiber supplements can rapidly produce dramatic and distressing changes. I know this from personal experience. Our local grocery store offered samples of a new fiber bar and a coupon to buy one and get one free. We returned home with two boxes. One April morning, I ate two of the 40-gram bars. Later that morning, I was overcome by intense diarrhea—so bad that I took anti-diarrhea medication and wondered whether I might be too sick to travel to a conference the next day. In trying to sort out whether I had food poisoning or a violent gastrointestinal bug or was having a strong reaction to what seemed like a harmless fiber supplement, I did an online search. I was one of *many* people who had an extreme reaction to this fiber supplement. All of us had made the same mistake of eating more than one bar. I described it to my husband because I wasn't going to eat any more of the bars, I didn't think our children should eat them, and I wanted to warn him against eating more than one serving at a time. But we had two boxes, and he figured that my reaction was unique or that I might be exaggerating for effect. I wasn't. He experienced intense cramping and even worse diarrhea that knocked him out for the better part of a day.

As suggested by my personal anecdote, laxatives, regardless of type, can cause bloating, cramping, and diarrhea. Laxative abuse has been associated with chronic or nocturnal diarrhea, constipation, bloody stool and rectal bleeding, pelvic floor dysfunction, abdominal tenderness, and darkening of the stomach (*gastric melanosis*) and colon (*melanosis coli*). Prolonged use can cause electrolyte imbalances, including reduced blood levels of sodium, potassium, magnesium, chloride, and blood bicarbonate, and laxative dependence.

Laxative dependence occurs when the body's chemistry shifts to counteract the effects of the laxative, leaving a person unable to have a bowel movement without using laxatives. These same shifts trigger water retention when laxatives are discontinued. One woman shared, "I have tried stopping my laxative abuse cold turkey, but it always fails. It's like my body doesn't know what to do after I quit taking laxatives and I bloat up so badly—put on 5–7 pounds in one day just from water weight. The last time I tried it was so bad that I could hardly bend my legs b/c they were so puffy from fluids. I ultimately had to start back on the laxatives b/c I could not stand it and hated the way I looked, etc." In her message, she described herself as hiding a "laxative addiction" for the past 12 years of her life, taking up to 60 per day.

Laxative abuse was identified as a cause of a specific type of kidney stone (*ammonium acid urate renal calculi*), answering a question posed by one woman, "I have also had numerous kidney stones which is making me wonder if my laxative abuse is causing this." Unfortunately, she also shared that "I have not told anybody about my laxative abuse, so therefore, I've never gotten the help needed."

Longer duration of laxative abuse contributes to worse kidney function. Laxative abuse may also increase the risk of developing kidney damage related to using pain medications.

COMPLICATIONS FROM DIURETIC MISUSE

Diuretics act on the kidneys to increase urination. Similar to laxatives, diuretics alter biological functions in different ways to produce this effect, and the medical consequences of diuretic abuse are linked to how they work. Most reports of severe medical consequences of diuretic abuse have emerged from patients taking prescription diuretics. Briefly, abuse of thiazides and the loop diuretic furosemide cause dehydration, potassium depletion, sodium depletion, decreased acidity of blood (*metabolic alkalosis*), and increased uric acid levels in the blood (*hyperuricemia*). Thiazides also contribute to increased blood calcium levels (*hypercalcemia*) whereas furosemide causes calcium depletion (*hypocalcemia*). In contrast to the effects of thiazides and furosemide, abuse of amiloride and triamterene increases acidity of blood (*metabolic acidosis*) and increases potassium levels (*hyperkalemia*). With this, you can see that some diuretics cause a loss of potassium whereas others cause an increase in potassium; however, both *too much* potassium and *too little* potassium contribute to irregular heartbeat. Because of their mechanisms of action, prescription diuretics can cause severe electrolyte imbalances that impair muscle function (including *hypokalemic paralysis*) and nerve function (including dysfunction of the central nervous system), and can lead to a heart attack, coma, or death. Diuretic abuse has been linked to a buildup of calcium deposits in the kidneys (*nephrocalcinosis*) and swelling in kidney tubules responsible for filtering fluids extracted from blood (*tubulointerstitital nephritis*). Both have been linked to kidney failure in eating disorders.

Based on accessibility, most individuals who abuse diuretics use either over-the-counter or herbal agents. Indeed, while walking through a charming country store in Helen, Georgia, my eye was drawn to a display of glass jars above an array of trivets to one labeled, "Diet Assist Herbal Tea" (Figure 6.2). Upon closer inspection, I found ingredients that act as diuretics. Herbal agents, like the one I found in a folksy jar, include a combination of dandelion (*Taraxacum officinale*), uva ursi, and juniper and increase urination and reduce inflammation. Many over-the-counter options include caffeine as the active agent to produce increased urination and magnesium salicylate to reduce inflammation. When used as directed and over short periods of time (less than one month), the FDA has judged these agents to be reasonably safe. However, in the context of purging, they aren't used as directed. The active ingredient in dandelion has been linked to increased calcium levels in the blood and increased heart rate, and the active ingredient in uva ursi has been linked to liver damage, eye damage (*retinal thinning*), breathing problems, and convulsions. Excess caffeine intake contributes to increased anxiety, insomnia, problems with diarrhea or gastric reflux, muscle breakdown, and increased blood pressure.

(a)

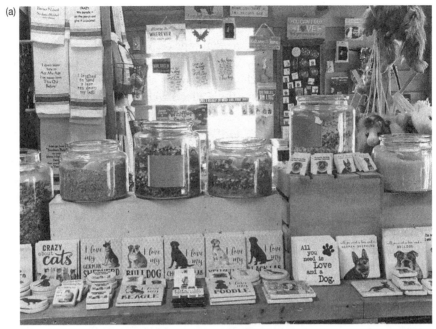

(b)

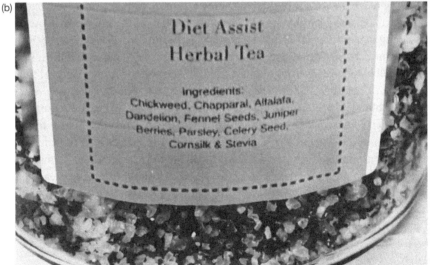

Figure 6.2 A country store sells a "Diet Assist Herbal Tea" that contains diuretics.

COMPLICATIONS FROM MISUSE OF THYROID MEDICATION AND INSULIN

Purging disorder can emerge in individuals taking medications for other conditions such as hypothyroidism or insulin-dependent diabetes mellitus. Prior to diagnosis, each of these diseases directly impacts metabolism and weight, and effective treatment largely reverses these effects. In the case of hypothyroidism, prior to diagnosis and treatment, individuals experience low mood, mood swings, fatigue, and weight gain, among other symptoms. The treatment for hypothyroidism is a manmade hormone that replaces what the thyroid gland isn't producing (levothyroxine sodium, found in Synthroid). This increases metabolism while reducing appetite, which may lead to weight loss. Some patients abuse their thyroid medication to enhance these effects. Side effects of thyroid medication misuse include nervousness, insomnia, and anxiety. Severe side effects include high blood pressure, irregular heartbeat, bone loss (*osteoporosis*), and heart failure (*cardiac failure*).

Type 1 diabetes (also known as insulin-dependent diabetes mellitus) typically develops in childhood or adolescence. Prior to diagnosis, individuals lose weight because their bodies do not produce insulin. Insulin is required to transport sugar from the blood into cells to be used for energy. To compensate, their bodies turn to body fat as a source of energy, which causes the weight loss. In addition, because the sugar from digested food builds up to excessive levels in the blood, the kidneys work to eliminate it through increasing urination. This causes additional weight loss due to dehydration. After beginning insulin treatment, insulin actively transports sugar that is broken down from food into cells for energy. Weight loss is rapidly reversed through rehydration. Indeed, some patients may experience swelling (*edema*) as their bodies adjust to retaining fluids that had been expelled along with excess sugar by their kidneys. Individuals with diabetes may purge by reducing or omitting insulin to force their bodies to burn fat for energy. Insulin omission increases sugar levels in blood (*hyperglycemia*), which damages nerves and small blood vessels throughout the body. Over time, this can lead to blindness (*retinopathy*), kidney failure (*nephropathy*), severe nerve damage (*neuropathy*), reduced blood flow, increased blood pressure (*hypertension*), heart disease (collectively referred to as *cardiovascular disease*), stroke, and amputation of extremities (e.g., feet) due to loss of blood flow. A byproduct of burning fat for energy use is high concentrations of ketonic acid in the blood (*ketoacidosis*). This is where the "keto diet" gets its name. Ketoacidosis causes extreme fatigue, nausea, uncontrollable vomiting, and shortness of breath. This represents a medical emergency requiring hospitalization because it can cause coma, brain damage, and death.

WHAT PHYSICIANS SHOULD LOOK FOR

According to the third edition of the Academy for Eating Disorder's *Guide to Medical Care*,[2] physical exams should include objective measures of height and weight, oral temperature, and lying and standing heart rate and blood pressure. In addition, a complete blood count should be ordered to evaluate for possible low white blood cell count (*leukopenia*), low red blood cell count (*anemia*), and low blood platelet count (*thrombocytopenia*). A comprehensive panel should include electrolytes, kidney function tests, and liver enzyme tests. High blood creatinine or urea nitrogen levels indicate possible kidney damage, and elevated blood urea nitrogen may also be a sign of heart failure. Urine specimens may be needed to determine presence of protein (*proteinuria*), blood (*hematuria*), or white blood cells (*leukocytes*), all of which indicate possible kidney injury or reduced kidney function to filter blood. Pending findings on electrolyte balance and lying and standing heart rate, an electrocardiogram should be used to check for potential cardiac arrhythmia.

If the clinical exam suggests possible softening of the bones due to frequent broken bones, muscle weakness, or pain, particularly in the hip bones, laboratory tests for low levels of vitamin D may indicate risk for poor bone health. Additional indicators include low calcium levels and decreasing phosphate levels. An X-ray may reveal small cracks in bone, and, very rarely, a bone biopsy may be used to diagnose bone softening. A bone mineral density test is the standard evaluation to determine whether bones have become soft or more porous.

If tests reveal that a patient is medically unstable, then hospitalization for acute medical stabilization should be instituted. After fainting, hitting her head on a table, and vomiting, Nicole Johns called a cab to take her to the emergency room because she feared she had a concussion. Tests revealed dehydration, electrolyte imbalances, and low blood pressure that dropped when she stood up. This contributed to her fainting because her body was unable to get sufficient blood to her brain to deliver oxygen. She was admitted to the cardiac unit for irregular heartbeat characterized by a slow heart rate; extra, abnormal heartbeats from the upper chamber of her heart (*premature atrial contractions*); and extra, abnormal heartbeats from the lower chamber of her heart (*premature ventricular contractions*). Even if initial tests indicate no medical complications, a physician should provide ongoing medical monitoring and care. Therapy does not immediately eliminate symptoms, and complications requiring medical intervention could emerge during treatment.

Although several of the complications related to purging may be managed by a primary care physician or generalist, some complications require consultation with specialists. A cardiologist may be needed to treat problems related to the heart. A gastroenterologist may be needed to address problems with constipation due to excessive laxative use, abdominal pain and nausea, blood in vomit (*hematemesis*), frequent heartburn, and early or excessive satiety. A nephrologist may be needed to address potential kidney disease.

Finally, patients with recurrent vomiting should receive ongoing dental care. From e-mails I've received over the years, dental problems are the most frequently described. Although the best way to prevent these problems is to stop purging, dental professionals can guide patients toward best practices to minimize the impact of purging on their mouths, gums, and teeth.

Those diagnosed with hypothyroidism or type 1 diabetes should be seen by an endocrinologist who may be the first to notice signs of purging through medication misuse. The primary method to reverse medical complications is to discontinue medication misuse. However, the consequences of medication misuse may require immediate treatment through either intensive outpatient or inpatient care and should involve medical and mental health professionals working within a coordinated treatment team.

This chapter specifically focuses on the known medical consequences of purging. For anyone using this behavior to control weight to be "healthier," this chapter fully refutes any notion that purging could make anyone healthier. For anyone questioning whether their purging is a problem and trying to decide whether they should get treatment, this chapter should eliminate uncertainty. It's not intended to guide self-diagnosis. Only a physician can perform tests to identify medical complications, offer treatment to support physical health, and provide referrals to specialists as needed.

I hope that none of what I've described is happening to you or to anyone you know. My goal for this chapter is to reduce the likelihood that these problems will occur and to minimize their impact by encouraging those with purging disorder, or purging in the context of any eating disorder, to seek medical care. Early detection and intervention are key to successful outcomes. I'm also hoping this information could help at least some people to stop purging. One woman wrote that electrolyte imbalances motivated her decision to stop purging. She still struggled with feeling fat but had promised never to return to laxatives or use diuretics because purging left her feeling terrible all the time. Another woman wrote, "Over the past 4 months (after I started throwing up blood) I have been coming to terms with my disorder, and seeking treatment." The next chapter focuses on seeking treatment.

MEDICAL TERMS AND THEIR MEANING

Ammonium acid urate renal calculi—specific type of kidney stone with high concentrations of ammonium and urate linked to laxative abuse
Anemia—low red blood cell count
Bradycardia—slow heartbeat
Buccal surfaces—sides of teeth by cheeks
Capillaries—small blood vessels
Cardiac arrest—heart attack when the heart suddenly stops beating
Cardiac arrythmia—irregular heartbeat
Cardiac failure—chronic condition in which the heart muscle is weakened and less able to pump blood and oxygen through the body, also known as congestive heart failure
Cardiovascular disease—reduced blood flow due to narrowed or blocked blood vessels that causes increased blood pressure, also known as heart disease
Cathartic colon—inability to completely empty the bowels resulting in bloating, a feeling of fullness, and abdominal pain
Colorectal cancer—cancer in the colon and rectum
Dehydration—severe loss of fluids in the body
Dental caries—cavities in teeth
Dentin—tooth layer below enamel
Edema—swelling or accumulation of excess fluid
Esophageal sphincter—contracting ring of muscle between the esophagus and stomach
Esophageal tears—tear in the lining of the esophagus
Esophagus—tube of muscles that takes food from the back of the throat to the stomach

Facial petechial hemorrhages—bleeding from small blood vessels on the face

Gastric artery rupture—tear in the blood vessel that carries blood from the heart to the stomach

Gastric melanosis—darkening of the stomach lining

Gastroesophageal intussusception—condition in which a portion of the stomach slides into the esophagus

Gastroesophageal reflux—involuntary return of stomach contents up the esophagus

Gastrosplenic ligament (tear of)—a tear of the tissue that is part of the greater omentum and connects the stomach to the spleen

Gingival recession—receding gums

Gingivitis—inflamed or irritated gums

Greater omentum (tear of)—a tear in the membrane that attaches the stomach to the back abdominal wall

Halitosis—bad breath

Haustral folds (loss of)—damage to the muscles and nerves of the colon causing it to lose its segmented appearance

Hematemesis—presence of blood in vomit

Hematuria—presence of blood in urine

Hepatic failure—liver failure

Hiatal hernia—condition in which the upper portion of the stomach pushes through the muscle separating the abdomen from the chest

Hyoid bone fracture—break in the bone that attaches the tongue to the throat

Hypercalcemia—increased calcium in the blood

Hyperglycemia—high blood sugar

Hyperkalemia—increased potassium in the blood

Hypertension—high blood pressure

Hyperuricemia—increased uric acid in the blood

Hypocalcemia—decreased calcium in the blood

Hypokalemia—low potassium in the blood

Hypokalemic paralysis—loss of muscle function due to low potassium levels

Hyponatremia—low sodium in the blood

Hypotension—low blood pressure

Ketoacidosis—increase in ketonic acid in the blood due to burning of fat stores

Laryngopharyngeal reflux—condition in which acid from the stomach comes up to the throat

Larynx—the "voice box" where the vocal cords are located; muscular air passage to lungs involved in breathing, producing sound, and protecting the trachea against inhaling food

Leukocytes (in urine)—presence of white blood cells in urine

Leukopenia—low white blood cell count

Mallory-Weiss tears—tear in the tissue of the lower esophagus where it meets the stomach

Melanosis coli—darkening of the colon lining

Metabolic acidosis—increased acidity of blood

Metabolic alkalosis—decreased acidity of blood

Necrotizing sialometaplasia—death of tissue that makes saliva

Nephrocalcinosis—buildup of calcium deposits in the kidneys

Nephropathy—kidney disease caused by damage to the small blood vessels

Neuropathy—severe damage to nerves leading to numbness or pain

Occlusal surfaces—biting surface of teeth

Osteomalacia—softening of the bones

Osteoporosis—loss of bone density in which the bone becomes more porous and more easily broken

Palatal surfaces—inside surface of teeth that faces the palate

Parotid sialadenosis—swelling of the glands near the cheeks that make saliva

Perioral erythema—reddening around the mouth

Pharynx—area at the back of the throat, behind the mouth and nasal cavity, and above the esophagus and larynx

Pneumonia—infection of the air sacs in the lungs

Premature atrial contractions—extra, abnormal heartbeats from the upper chamber of the heart

Premature ventricular contractions—extra, abnormal heartbeats from the lower chamber of the heart

Proteinuria—presence of protein in urine

Rectal prolapse—protrusion of the rectum through the anus

Renal failure—condition in which the kidneys stop working

Retinal thinning—thinning of the back of the eye that can lead to blindness

Retinopathy—damage to the retina in the back of the eye due to abnormal blood flow

Retrosternal burning—heartburn

Rhabdomyolysis—breakdown of muscle tissue and release of contents into the bloodstream

Sialomegaly—swelling of saliva glands

Squamous cell carcinoma (of the esophagus)—cancer in the small flat cells that line the esophagus

Subconjunctival hemorrhages—broken blood vessel in the eye

Tachycardia—fast heart rate (more than 100 beats per minute)

Telangiectasia—condition in which small blood vessels widen, creating the appearance of fine threads or spiderwebs on skin ("spider veins")

Temporary facial purpura—rash of purple spots on the face caused by burst small vessels in skin that fade with time

Thrombocytopenia—low blood platelet count

Getting Help

There is a vast chasm between the number of people suffering from purging disorder and the number getting treatment. This chapter describes systemic barriers to eating disorders treatment, and advocacy will be needed to increase access to and decrease the cost of treatment for all eating disorders. This chapter also covers barriers that appear to uniquely impact purging disorder, making it invisible to those charged with providing care. I break down the levels of care available and what should happen when a person seeks treatment to support those ready to get help. This chapter is also intended to help clinicians recognize purging disorder when they see it. Otherwise, clinicians may assign symptoms that aren't present to make a patient fit what they know. This is another way that purging disorder remains invisible. Information on resources for patients, caregivers, and treatment providers is offered in the Additional Resources section at the end of this book.

The first step in getting a treatment that works is getting treatment. Yes, that seems obvious, but most people with purging disorder never seek any treatment for their illness. Why not? For one, many aren't sure their purging is a problem. One man wrote, "Even after a normal meal I will feel uncomfortable and must throw up." This was his life for 10 years, yet he added, "I am in excellent health and am comfortable living like this, even though I would rather not." This acceptance of regular purging as a normal part of life rather than as an eating disorder is reflected in findings from a large sample of Australian teens. This study identified 146 kids with purging disorder. Of these, 27 did not report significant distress or impairment despite purging at least weekly. In comparison, for the 206 teens with bulimia, all expressed at least moderate distress. Distress was missing in more kids with purging disorder than with any other eating disorder, suggesting that purging in the absence of binge eating and underweight may not be seen as a "real" problem. This may partially explain why purging disorder is relatively rare in treatment settings.

Among inpatients, the ratio of patients with bulimia to purging disorder is almost 10:1, and the ratio for anorexia to purging disorder patients is almost 17:1.

Among outpatients, those with anorexia outnumber purging disorder patients by 7:1, and patients with bulimia outnumber purging disorder patients by almost 6:1. Although distress may explain part of why purging disorder isn't seen in eating disorder programs, it can't fully explain the underrepresentation of purging disorder in treatment. Returning to that study of Australian teens, when diagnoses were restricted to those who endorsed severe distress, impairment, or both, the ratio of bulimia to purging disorder was 2:1 and the ratio of anorexia to purging disorder was 1:3.

Even if someone with purging disorder isn't bothered by their behaviors, the body still suffers the consequences. One woman shared how she had purged for 22 years, and "I don't think of this as a disorder" and "I have never felt the need to see a doctor for this." Yet she also acknowledged that "my right index finger started to show signs of stomach acid." Another woman wrote, "I am currently normal weight but I vomit 6-10 times a day after eating a meal. I know I am not bulimic and am not planning on visiting a doctor about it but it bothers me a little" and added that she had "major dental problems." By the time those with purging disorder seek treatment, they are likely to be older and more medically compromised. This hurts their chances for a successful treatment outcome.

Not seeking treatment for purging disorder contributes to a second factor that reduces the likelihood of recovery for those who *do* seek treatment. When only one out of six people seeking eating disorders treatment have purging disorder, clinicians can't get as much experience treating purging disorder as they do for other eating disorders. This decreases clinicians' ability, and perhaps willingness, to recognize purging disorder for what it is. Over and over, people described being told they had an eating disorder they knew they didn't have. As one wrote, "I have been in counseling for years and they tell me that I have bulimia nervosa. I tell them that I do not over eat. I would perge [sic] at will, even if I ate a small meal." And another wrote, "For more then [sic] 20 yrs. I struggled with this. No one would listen they just wanted to put me into one or the other category." Another shared, "I have—since about 13-14 years old—been what doctors call bulimic—but I never binge and I cant [sic] even eat a normal meal without feeling the need to purge just to not feel so uncomfortable." If the clinician's toolbox only has treatments for anorexia or bulimia, everything starts looking like anorexia or bulimia. To break this harmful cycle, more people with purging disorder need to seek treatment, and clinicians need to recognize purging disorder for what it is and adapt treatment approaches to the specific problems associated with it.

The first step in seeking treatment is participating in an intake assessment. Although assessment can have therapeutic benefits, its goals are to establish an eating disorder diagnosis, symptom severity, presence of medical complications, related mental health concerns, and readiness to change. Assessment may or may not be conducted by the person who will provide treatment because clinicians can't be sure how to help someone until they know what kind of help the person needs. Intake assessments guide development of a treatment plan, which includes decisions about level of care needed.

LEVELS OF CARE

Levels of care include inpatient units, residential treatment programs (also referred to as rehabilitation centers), day or evening programs (also referred to as
partial hospital programs), and outpatient clinics. Each level provides a different
intensity of care. Levels of care also differ in terms of cost and accessibility.

Both inpatient and residential treatment programs provide the most intensive level of care because patients live in their treatment facility, with 24/7 access to nursing staff, as well as frequent on-site contact with dietitians, therapists,
and physicians. The availability of inpatient eating disorder programs differs
across the United States and around the globe because they are typically offered
in university-affiliated hospitals. Outside of these university-affiliated inpatient
programs, a lot of inpatient treatment occurs on adolescent or adult psychiatric or
medical wards that don't specialize on eating disorders.

The high intensity of care translates into high costs. Based on insurance claims
data collected in 1995 in the United States, inpatient treatment for an eating disorder cost $599 per day (and that was 25 years ago as of this writing). Due to
their high costs, inpatient treatment in the United States is reserved for acute
medical and psychiatric stabilization with the duration of care limited to the time
needed to permit safe transfer of the patient to a less intense level of care. Based
on these same insurance claims data, patients spent an average of 20 days in inpatient treatment for an average cost of $12,155 in 1995. Importantly, this does not
necessarily reflect 20 consecutive days because some patients may have had repeated hospitalizations over the 12-month period. Given the rising costs of health
care, it's likely that inpatient treatment for eating disorders costs a great deal more
now than it did in 1995. More recent studies have examined overall health care
costs (vs. services specifically to treat an eating disorder) and report the economic
burden at a societal level (i.e., annual health care costs to the United States or to
Canada for those with eating disorders). These data are important to public policy
makers but don't easily translate into what inpatient treatment costs.

Residential eating disorder treatment programs have become increasingly
common in the United States over the last three decades to fill the gap between
those needing more intensive specialized care and beds available on inpatient
units. Residential programs offer a longer duration of treatment, with a mean
length of stay of 83 days. Nicole Johns' *Rehab Diaries* provides a first-hand account of her experience in a Wisconsin residential treatment program, where she
stayed for 88 days. Her program, like many others, had a floor dedicated to eating
disorders and provided rehabilitation services for other conditions on other floors
(for example, support for addictions). A 2006 study surveyed residential treatment
program directors on eating disorder program costs. Across the 19 programs who
responded, the mean cost was $956 per day, for a total cost of $79,348 per patient.
Again, it's likely that current costs exceed $30,000 per month. Indeed, during my
office hours, a student recently shared that she volunteered at a local residential
center for eating disorders that charged $40,000 per month of treatment. These

costs limit residential treatment programs to those with good insurance coverage or more financial resources. To help with the high costs of care, nonprofit organizations in the United States have developed scholarship programs to support the cost of residential treatment for those who can't afford it.[1]

Day or evening programs provide an intermediate intensity of care and are often offered as a transition from inpatient/residential to outpatient treatment. This limits their availability to places that have an inpatient or residential program for eating disorders. Patients sleep in their own homes or a local extended-stay hotel and during the day or evening come to the treatment facility, where they receive group and individual therapy and support in eating at least two meals and snacks without restricting or purging. Evening programs are compatible with working a full-time day job for those who live near a partial hospital program. And evenings cover unstructured time when many patients find it most difficult to manage their symptoms.

Outpatient treatment is the least intensive, most common, and least expensive level of care. Costs depend on where you live (outpatient sessions cost more in large cities than in smaller towns), who you see (psychiatrists cost more than psychologists who cost more than clinical social workers), and how often you attend sessions. Based on 1995 insurance claims data, eating disorder patients received an average of 15 "days" (probably sessions) of outpatient treatment with an average total cost of $1,826, or $123 per visit. In addition to being lower than current treatment costs, these numbers may reflect negotiated rates with the insurance companies. Without insurance, a patient may expect to pay $20 to $250 for a 50-minute session with a licensed therapist.

Given the differences in access and cost, it's reasonable to question the benefits associated with each level of care. A comparison of generalized outpatient treatment, specialized outpatient treatment, and specialized inpatient treatment suggested that there was an equivalent likelihood of recovery from anorexia at one year. In addition, specialized outpatient treatment offered both a lower cost for care and higher patient satisfaction. This means that a lot can be accomplished by working with the most available option, outpatient care, using a treatment tailored for eating disorders. There are some important caveats to this conclusion, however. Findings were based on treatment of anorexia in adolescents who were safe to be seen on an outpatient basis, and results come from the United Kingdom. Results aren't relevant for those who require a higher level of care to ensure their safety, and we can only hope findings extend to the treatment of *purging disorder* in adolescents *and adults* in the United Kingdom *and beyond*. That might be a lot to hope for.

Speaking of the United Kingdom, the National Health Service covers the cost of specialized eating disorder treatment for everyone receiving a referral from their general practitioner (GP). However, the number of patients needing treatment far exceeds the number of trained providers, creating delays between referral and receiving treatment. As one woman shared on her Twitter account, "I'm on the waiting list. I'm waiting. No matter how many times I speak to my GP, it's not going to reduce the waiting time for treatment. #eatingdisorders," and "I literally

CANNOT do any more but wait, unless someone wants to pay for private treatment. #MentalHealth in England."

To address these gaps, technology has entered the realm of treatment through telemedicine, online resources, and treatment apps for smartphones. In the United States, the National Eating Disorders Association (NEDA) offers a toll-free support line and online service to identify treatment options throughout the country. In the United Kingdom, Beat (short for Beat Eating Disorders) offers a helpline, online support groups, peer coaching, and resources for finding treatment. Additional options for help include self-help books and guided self-help. The key is that doing something is better than doing nothing, and seeking treatment through any of these resources is doing something. Similarly, participating in an intake assessment is doing something, even if it feels like a further delay in treatment.

ASSESSMENT

Chapter 6 outlined medical tests to evaluate potential consequences of purging. These should be done early in assessment to ensure that a patient is healthy enough for outpatient treatment. Otherwise, inpatient or residential treatment should be used for acute medical stabilization. In a study of 215 adolescent eating disorder patients admitted for medical complications (e.g., slow heart rate, low blood pressure, electrolyte imbalances), 95% experienced moderate to severe malnutrition even though nearly a third had a minimally healthy weight. An average of 11 days of inpatient treatment produced medical stability in this cohort. Briefly, patients had continuous heart monitoring in their rooms, at least daily checks of electrolytes, and dietary supplements of phosphorous, potassium, and magnesium as indicated by lab results. To address malnutrition, patients were initially placed on bed rest and given a daily caloric intake goal of 1,200 calories (or 500 calories above home intake, whichever was higher) consumed over three meals per day. Their metabolism and age were used to calculate a caloric goal for discharge. On average, patients consumed 1,466 calories per day at intake and 3,800 calories per day at discharge over three meals and two snacks per day because over two-thirds of these patients were underweight. Importantly, a lower calorie goal was accepted for patients who regularly purged, and they were monitored after every meal to prevent purging.

Objective measures of height and weight, along with age and gender for minors, indicate whether weight falls above a minimally healthy threshold to rule out a diagnosis of anorexia. For adults, a BMI of 18.5 kg/m^2 suggests a minimally normal weight for height. For adolescents, a BMI above the fifth percentile for age and biological sex (that is, greater than the lowest 5% of the person's same-sex peers) suggests a minimally normal weight.[2] Importantly, these represent *guidelines*, not hard-and-fast rules. If a physician determines that a patient is medically underweight, then weight gain will be a focus of treatment, and a diagnosis of anorexia or possibly avoidant restrictive food intake disorder may be warranted. Resources are available to guide treatment for these eating disorders, including the threshold for instituting inpatient treatment for safe weight restoration (see Additional Resources at the end of the book).

Assessment should evaluate eating episodes when a patient feels any loss of control over eating and the amount of food consumed during those episodes. If the amount is definitely larger than what most people would eat under similar circumstances, then a diagnosis of bulimia or subthreshold bulimia may be warranted, and readily available treatment guides for bulimia should be followed. Even though episodes won't be large for patients with purging disorder by definition (see chapter 1), the frequency of loss of control over eating is linked to greater patient distress and impairment. This makes it an important treatment target. In addition, it's likely to trigger purging. Helping patients regain a sense of control over their eating will help them stop purging.

If there is no loss of control when eating or if food intake is *not* definitely larger than what most people would eat, then most standardized interviews direct assessors to skip the remaining questions, including questions about purging. Both the Structured Clinical Interview for DSM-5 Mental Disorders (SCID-5) and the World Health Organization Composite International Diagnostic Interview (WHO CIDI) instruct interviewers to skip questions about purging in individuals who aren't underweight and don't have large binge episodes. But questions about purging *should not be skipped*. This represents a serious flaw in these assessments based on the false premise that diagnostic criteria capture everything of clinical interest and that a huge amount of time will be saved by not asking irrelevant questions.

We examined the impact of following versus not following the skip rules for the SCID and found that 6 out of 10 people who purged to control their weight would be missed by following skip rules. Also, it took only *two extra minutes* to ask all of the questions that would have been skipped. Bottom line: Every eating disorder assessment should *always* ask about purging. (If I had my way, every assessment of mental illness would ask about purging.)

When clinicians ask about purging, it's important to understand the context in which purging occurs. Sometimes patients describe their vomiting as involuntary instead of self-induced, and this can create ambiguity about whether there is an underlying medical condition causing vomiting or whether the vomiting is part of an eating disorder (vs. a somatoform disorder; see chapter 2). In addition, involuntary vomiting may occur when gastroesophageal reflux develops as a complication of self-induced vomiting (see chapter 6). If vomiting occurs in private settings and never occurs in public (for example, when a patient is on public transportation or in the middle of a meeting), then patients have some control over their vomiting. For these patients, the experience of vomiting as involuntary may reflect the strength of the compulsion to purge. Clinicians should ask about the duration and frequency of purging behaviors, including the daily, weekly, or monthly frequency of self-induced vomiting, laxative use, enema use, and diuretic use to control weight as well as the frequency of any other extreme weight control behaviors, such as fasting, excessive or compulsive exercise, and misuse of other medications. A shorter duration of purging before treatment tends to improve chances of recovery because fewer medical complications will have developed and it won't be as entrenched in the person's life. I don't think it's a coincidence that many of the people who indicated that their purging wasn't a problem had been doing it for 10 or more years of their lives. For these individuals, purging felt more normal than not purging. Both the number of different purging methods and purging frequency indicate severity because they increase the likelihood for medical complications. For those who purge multiple times per day using multiple methods, inpatient or residential treatment may be needed to break the cycle. For Johns, both the intensity of her purging (at least five days a week, up to multiple times per day) and its severe medical consequences (heart problems, low blood pressure, and electrolyte imbalances) necessitated intensive care, and her health care insurance covered 100% of the cost of her residential treatment program, which totaled $24,500.

After ruling out diagnoses of anorexia and bulimia, purging disorder is the right diagnosis for those who purge after consuming normal amounts of food and who are not underweight. An additional diagnosis of atypical anorexia may be warranted if the patient has recently lost a substantial amount of weight. There are no rules against diagnosing both purging disorder and atypical anorexia if both conditions fit. We find that individuals with purging disorder typically weigh less than their highest prior weight. In our most recent study, participants with purging disorder weighed approximately 12 lbs (5.6 kg) less than their highest lifetime weight. At least part of this is related to dehydration from purging, and part is due to their other weight loss efforts. As covered in chapter 1, individuals with purging disorder are deeply invested in avoiding fat. This motivates their purging, and it motivates other extreme weight control behaviors, including restricting the types and quantities of food they eat, sometimes to the point of fasting, and exercising excessively. At admission, Johns weighed 133 lbs, 27 lbs less than her highest weight of 160 lbs nine months before. These behaviors, combined with weight loss, are captured in a diagnosis of atypical anorexia. The value of adding a diagnosis of atypical anorexia depends on whether treatment has a goal of increasing weight or weight trajectory. At intake, Johns' weight fell within the target range of 127 to 140 set by her dietitian. This means that gaining weight was not a treatment goal, and she could even lose a little bit of weight without causing concern, but they didn't want her BMI to drop below 21 kg/m^2.

The program at Children's Hospital of Philadelphia emphasizes a non–weight-biased approach to treatment. They examine patients' growth charts prior to diagnosis, and unless the child's weight was extremely underweight or overweight, they help patients return to their previous growth trajectory. They focus on growth trajectory because children are supposed to gain weight with age. Their goal is to get kids back on track with their own developmental trajectory. This approach is non–weight-biased because it acknowledges and accepts a wide range of weights as healthy for a given height, age, and gender. Remember that children who later developed purging disorder had histories of higher BMI percentiles compared to those who didn't develop eating disorders. This could mean that, for these children, a higher weight is a healthier weight. Rather than expecting everyone to fall at the middle of the healthy weight range, the non–weight-biased approach accepts higher BMI percentiles as healthy. This contrasts with the approach taken in Johns' residential program, in which her BMI was expected to fall between 21 and 23.5 kg/m², a far more narrow range than defined as healthy by the U.S. Centers for Disease Control and Prevention. In other research, we've found that a larger difference between highest previous weight and current weight is linked to longer illness duration across eating disorders, including purging disorder. This suggests that weight gain may facilitate recovery even when patients aren't underweight. In these instances, the additional diagnosis of atypical anorexia may help capture the value of supporting weight gain as healthy even among those who aren't underweight. Importantly, a diagnosis of bulimia precludes a diagnosis of atypical anorexia, no matter how much weight patients have lost from their highest weight. Similarly, among those with atypical anorexia who purge, a diagnosis of purging disorder remains valuable because purging still has to be addressed in treatment. Patients who stop restricting their food intake and gain weight won't be considered recovered if they're still purging.

RELATED MENTAL HEALTH PROBLEMS

To produce recovery, treatment also may need to address related mental illnesses. Purging disorder often co-occurs with other emotional and behavioral problems, including, but not limited to, depression, anxiety, substance use, and suicidality. Across community-based, outpatient, and inpatient samples, depression affects approximately half of those with purging disorder. Anxiety disorders affect 1 in 4 and substance use disorders affect 1 in 10 individuals with purging disorder. In forming a treatment plan, it's critical to determine how the eating disorder is related to other mental health problems. In many cases, there are problems with mood and anxiety that contribute to and result from purging behavior. In addition, certain factors, such as perfectionism, body dissatisfaction, and interpersonal conflict, may serve as risk and maintenance factors across the different disorders. This can create uncertainty about what to address first. The following case study illustrates this point.[3]

Elizabeth was a college student who sought treatment for anxiety. During intense bouts of anxiety, she would physically damage her body. More often, she took laxatives to feel better. She had started taking laxatives after a teammate in gymnastics teased Elizabeth about her weight. Elizabeth's anxiety peaked when she checked her body for fat—a ritual of pinching and poking her body that began when she first started competing in gymnastics. Now she used laxatives daily to manage her anxiety and her weight and to make it possible to have a bowel movement. She found that she needed to take more and more laxatives to get the empty feeling to calm her fears of being fat. Fears she maintained despite having a body weight in the healthy range for her height.

Dialectical behavior therapy organizes a patient's problems into a hierarchy to guide what to tackle first. At the top of the hierarchy are problems that are life threatening or threaten safety, followed by those that interfere with therapy, followed by those that are distressing and interfere with a patient's ability to function. In Elizabeth's case, her anxiety was highly distressing, but purging has a host of medical consequences, and she was already demonstrating laxative dependence, making it a more imminent threat to her safety. In addition, her assessment suggested that her fear of fat contributed to both her anxiety and laxative use, and that the anxiety triggered her non-suicidal self-harm. If treatment could successfully address the first two steps in this chain, fear of fat and laxative misuse, it might lessen anxiety and eliminate self-harm.

Often symptoms of other disorders improve dramatically along with eating disorder remission because purging exacerbates most problems. In a longitudinal follow-up study, those with diagnoses of purging disorder were 2.5 times more likely to go on to develop depression, almost four times more likely to develop anxiety disorders or substance use disorders, and almost five times more likely to begin engaging in self-harming behavior. For these individuals, successfully treating their purging disorder may have protected them from developing these other problems later on. Finally, the approaches and skills used to treat purging disorder can be transferred to address unresolved symptoms of other disorders because the interventions come from a broader class of treatments originally developed for depression and anxiety.

SUICIDE RISK

Although the decision to begin treatment for purging disorder before working on problems related to depression or anxiety depends on case conceptualization, other problems, such as suicide risk, will be at the top of any treatment hierarchy. You may have heard that eating disorders are the deadliest of any psychiatric illness. The leading cause of death in eating disorders isn't due to medical complications. It's suicide. One study examined public inpatient records to document hospitalizations for suicide attempts in Sweden. Approximately 1 out of 10 individuals with purging disorder had made at least one suicide attempt, making them 9 times more likely to attempt suicide that individuals with no eating disorder and 3 times more likely than those with restricting anorexia. On average, individuals with purging disorder made more than two suicide attempts, and 1 out of 4 attempts was categorized as violent (e.g., use of a gun, knife, or hanging). These numbers come from a population-based study. In a case series of eating disorder outpatients, one-third of purging disorder patients reported suicidal ideation, and approximately 1 in 6 had attempted suicide. For this reason, I'm going to delve into this topic in some detail.

For many patients, suicide risk can be managed on an outpatient basis through frequent assessment, a coping card to manage crises, and a safety contract. Frequent assessment can include having sessions twice a week with daily check-ins by phone between sessions. A coping card lists activities the patient will use to cope with increased urges for self-harm that are soothing and enjoyable, such as calling a friend, listening to music, or going for a walk. The card lists as many activities as the patient can think of, and the patient agrees to try all of those activities and do them again before acting on suicidal urges. This is embedded in a safety contract in which a patient commits to seeking help, including calling emergency services, before acting on any suicidal urges. Most people wouldn't hesitate to call 911 in the United States or 999 in the United Kingdom if their life was threatened by a house fire. Similarly, they should not hesitate to call emergency services if their lives are in danger due to their own urges. Emergency personnel are trained to help individuals in crises and can take them to emergency services for immediate psychiatric evaluations for possible inpatient care. For patients who cannot keep themselves safe from suicidal urges, inpatient treatment for psychiatric stabilization should be instituted immediately.

Although Cara entered treatment for an eating disorder, we spent most of our first six months focused on her suicidality. Using my training in dialectical behavior therapy, I had created a hierarchy of symptoms and behaviors that were life threatening, followed by those that interfered with therapy, followed by those that were distressing and interfered with Cara's ability to function. Her desire to commit suicide represented an imminent risk to her life that took precedence over the purging as our treatment focus. I checked in with her weekly on her weight and purging symptoms, and she continued seeing her doctor to monitor her electrolyte levels and vital signs to ensure her medical stability. However, very little of our therapy focused on changing her eating disorder symptoms. Instead, we focused on lowering her risk for suicide. Cara believed the world would be a better place without her. She didn't believe that she had any value, felt exhausted by her own cycle of purging and restricting, and expressed minimal aversion to dying. Her multiple piercings and tattoos demonstrated that she also had little fear of pain. She had no prior suicide attempts but described her purging as an indirect attempt to kill herself.

Her suicide plan was to overdose on pills. She was smart and knew that taking too many of some over-the-counter medicines could be lethal. However, she had made no effort to obtain any medications for a suicide attempt. This was important because anything that delays a patient from acting on an urge creates an opportunity for the urge to pass and to get help. Had she been stockpiling pills, we would have needed to engage in means restriction. This involves restricting a patient's access to lethal means of attempting suicide. It can include a patient giving a firearm to a relative for safekeeping or using a gun lock, driving a route that avoids any bridges or overpasses, or flushing pills down a toilet, or, for patients who need to take prescription medications for other conditions, having the prescription changed or giving most of their pills to another to securely store so that they don't have access to enough to be life threatening. In each case, patients actively agree to limit their access to a method that could kill them.

Based on my assessment, Cara's desire for suicide was high, and she had a specific plan. But her intent to follow through was low, and she had made no prior attempts, she had no current means to make an attempt, and she agreed to engage in coping and reach out for support, including calling 911, before she would act on any suicidal urges. Her ability to keep herself safe was key to our ability to continue treatment on an outpatient basis.

During those first six months, we spent considerable time discussing the likely consequences of a suicide attempt. Although Cara wasn't afraid of pain or death, she was afraid that an attempt might leave her disabled instead of dead. Given that most suicide attempts do not cause death, I reinforced that her concerns were well founded. As part of my dissertation research, I had interviewed a woman who had tried to kill herself by drinking a lot of alcohol, pouring the remainder of the alcohol over her bedding, getting in bed, and lighting it on fire. She jumped out of the burning bed, and, years later, she was grateful she had survived and recovered from her eating disorder. However, she did live the rest of her life with scarring on her arm and face. Cara and I also discussed who would be affected by her death. When she claimed that no one would miss her, I asserted that I would be deeply affected and used that as evidence that she might not be accurately considering the true consequences for those who loved her. Slowly and steadily over the course of our sessions, Cara identified more reasons to live and more reasons not to kill herself. Once her desire for suicide abated to a manageable level—it was present but not pressing—we were able to move on to treating her purging disorder.

Other cases may involve trauma, manic episodes, or alcohol or drug abuse that must be addressed before it's possible to make headway in treating purging disorder. In cases of abuse, community-based resources can be enlisted to ensure that patients remain in a safe environment. For patients who are in a manic episode, initiation of medication in an inpatient unit may be needed to ensure therapeutic doses are reached and to protect patients from harming themselves or others. Similarly, outpatient treatment may be insufficient when there are concerns about withdrawal or inability to stop alcohol or drug use outside of a controlled setting. In such cases, inpatient or residential rehabilitation services should be used to ensure safety. As distressing as purging may be, purging disorder cannot be successfully treated in a patient who is manic, wasted, or dead. In Cara's case, once she committed to living, we could focus on her purging behavior.

AMBIVALENCE AND MOTIVATIONAL INTERVIEWING

In retrospect, I wish I had done a better job of assessing not only Cara's commitment to living but also her commitment to recovery. Ambivalence about treatment represents another major barrier for getting help. When I started seeing Cara, successful approaches for assessing treatment ambivalence were established for alcohol use disorder and were rapidly expanding to other mental health problems, but they hadn't quite reached the field of eating disorders. This strikes me as strange given that ambivalence was recognized as a major treatment barrier in eating disorders from the very beginning. In fact, the diagnostic criteria for anorexia codify ambivalence in defining the illness by including "persistent lack of recognition of the seriousness of the current low body weight."[4] For purging disorder, like anorexia, there can be a lack of recognition of the seriousness of purging. In describing her experiences in a residential program, one woman recounted how they had cameras in the room, sat with her while she ate, and followed her for an hour after meals to prevent her from purging. "I know, I should've been thankful but instead I was determined to keep control of what was mine." Three years later, she was still purging three or four times per day, adding, "it's like I want help but trying to train my body and my mind not to be one way is so much harder." It's not that people want to have purging disorder or don't want to recover, it's just that they're afraid of what recovery will cost them.

Ambivalence differs considerably across the eating disorders. Patients with large binge episodes, including those with bulimia and BED, experience higher levels of distress. Losing control and eating large amounts of food makes them feel bad about themselves and triggers fears about weight gain. Binge eating is also expensive, socially isolating, and time consuming. This distress increases motivation to stop binge eating, which explains higher treatment completion rates for bulimia compared to anorexia and purging disorder. In a large case series from Canada, 8 out of 10 patients with bulimia (80%) completed treatment compared to about 6 out of 10 patients with anorexia or purging disorder. Similar completion rates for purging disorder were reported in case series from Spain. Purging disorder cannot be successfully treated in a patient who does not fully engage in treatment or drops out prematurely. Motivational interviewing is a form of assessment designed to resolve ambivalence and should be incorporated in transitioning from assessment to treatment planning.

Motivational interviewing expands assessment's focus from what a person is doing to why they are doing it—specifically, what are the benefits of continuing to purge, what are the costs of purging, what are the benefits of recovery, and what are the costs of recovery? Answers to these and other questions establish a patient's readiness to change, which is divided into six sequential stages: precontemplation, contemplation, preparation, action, maintenance, and (successful) termination. For example, if precontemplation represents a person who is not even ready to acknowledge that they have a problem, then contemplation involves considering the possibility of talking to a health professional, preparation means finding a clinic, and action involves making the appointment and keeping it. This all reflects readiness to change and acknowledging that there may be a problem. The duration of each stage varies by person. Although a patient can't realistically skip steps moving forward (e.g., a patient can't skip from precontemplation to action), it's shockingly easy to skip stages in falling backwards (e.g., a patient can easily relapse from action to contemplation).

The questions and feedback on responses during motivational interviewing support patients in moving to the next stage. For example, a patient can decide to engage in a treatment plan or decide not to. One of my three patients with purging disorder at Massachusetts General Hospital completed her assessment and never returned. She had not come into the assessment of her own accord. Her older sister learned of her purging, insisted she see someone, and even drove her to the appointment. The patient was very clear that she was only meeting with me to appease her sister and did not want to be in treatment. If her sister hadn't waited for her in the waiting room, I'm not even sure she would have completed the assessment.

After starting treatment, a patient can decide to maintain the changes being made or not. Another patient with purging disorder started treatment, began eating regularly, and stopped vomiting. However, within three weeks, she found that she couldn't tolerate weight gain and terminated treatment.

Only Cara initiated and stayed in treatment. However, she continued to experience considerable ambivalence about purging. She wanted to get better, but she didn't want to get fat. Motivational interviewing might have helped Cara with her ambivalence and might have helped my other patients' motivation to follow through on treatment.

For those with purging disorder, change can be so frightening that it seems impossible. Convinced that something is fundamentally wrong with their bodies, many fear that any effort to give up purging will cause their bodies to run amok. It's important to bring these fears to light and address them head on. In these instances, it can be helpful to think back to a time before purging and reflect on their relationship to food and their bodies. This time often starkly contrasts with the present in its freedom from constant fear of what they put in their mouths and how they were going to keep from getting fat, freedom to eat with friends and eat what they wanted, and freedom from making excuses for trips to the bathroom. Generally, this freedom didn't feel out of control. How could they lose control over a body they weren't actively trying to control? Reflecting on a time when they were free of an eating disorder *and* felt fine about their bodies provides evidence that it's safe to hope for recovery.

Acknowledging they may gain weight with recovery and may need to wear a larger size in clothing opens a conversation about what that means in the context of their eating disorder versus what that would mean without an eating disorder. In the context of purging disorder, gaining 5 lbs (over 2 kg) feels like the start of a never-ending climb to morbid obesity. But what if, after gaining 5 lbs, they felt more comfortable in their own body because they knew that they were taking good care of themselves? Rather than just looking healthy on the outside, they could *be* healthy. For example, a motivational interviewer might observe, "So, it sounds like, right now, a 5-pound weight gain would be devastating. But, if you put your eating disorder behind you, you could be free of worrying about the number on the scale and focus on what makes you feel strong and healthy instead?" Motivational interviewers reinforce patients' own positive reasons for change and frame summaries as questions. This invites patients to elaborate or clarify their thinking. If the patient responds, "I don't think I could ever stop worrying about the number on the scale," then the motivational interviewer could ask, "So being completely free of that worry sounds unrealistic, but how do you think recovery would impact that worry?" Although the purpose of motivational interviewing is to resolve ambivalence and encourage change, the goal is *not* to win a debate. A patient's motivation to change is not subject to refutation. Instead, motivational interviewing helps patients see both sides of the decision they face and reinforces the side that motivates change—ergo, the name "motivational interviewing."

Although motivational interviewing has therapeutic value, it actually serves as a prelude and companion to treatment. Without specific agreed-upon goals to discontinue purging and a means to reach those goals, no amount of understanding readiness to change is going to magically produce that change. In addition, motivation to change is hard to maintain if no changes are made. As described in chapter 4, negative reinforcement is a powerful maintenance factor in purging disorder. Most patients purge to prevent a dreaded outcome, such as intolerable distress or becoming fat. As my college friend shared, she didn't vomit because it helped her lose weight; it just kept the weight off. In response to motivational interviewing, this would be an example of a reason to purge. Once you've purged, you can't know what would have happened if you hadn't purged. Without evidence to support or refute any conclusion, you can feel like purging got rid of your bad feelings and prevented weight gain. What's worse is that even if you feel awful after purging, you can still believe that it would have been much worse if you hadn't purged. The only way to challenge and change these beliefs is to change behaviors. When a patient stops purging during the treatment process, they experience the true consequences of not purging. Like most things, the consequences are neither all bad nor all good, making them more manageable than the consequences they imagined. Looking back at imagined costs that never actually occurred can reveal how much the illness creates barriers to getting healthy and why treatment is worth the effort. One of the greatest motivators for treatment is early improvement in treatment.

In fact, one study including patients with purging disorder in a partial hospitalization program found better outcomes for a form of cognitive-behavioral therapy emphasizing early change than for motivational interviewing followed by cognitive-behavioral therapy. Notably, a partial hospitalization program provides an intensive level of care in which patients willingly place themselves in a controlled environment for most of the day. Similar outcomes may or may not be found for outpatients.

TRANSITIONING FROM ASSESSMENT TO TREATMENT PLAN

For both patients and clinicians, it's important for assessment to lead to a treatment plan and to start treatment. Delays in treatment initiation can occur for several reasons, including the problems already described with access, costs, and ambivalence. An additional and avoidable source of delay comes from the belief that you must complete assessment before beginning treatment. On the face of it, this seems logical, but it's based on flawed logic. Although you have to *begin* assessment before you begin treatment, you don't have to *finish* assessment before you begin treatment. Instead, assessment should continue throughout treatment.

Treatment doesn't mark the end of assessment; it simply marks a transition in the function of assessment. Prior to treatment, assessment identifies the problem(s), the level of care needed, maintaining factors for the problem(s), motivation to change, and what treatments effectively reduce or eliminate those maintaining factors. Once patients make the transition to treatment, assessment continues to evaluate their readiness to change because treatment involves a series of changes. Ongoing assessment determines whether the intervention is being used, whether maintaining factors are changing, and whether symptoms and associated problems are decreasing and eventually eliminated. The next chapter covers what happens when treatment starts.

What Happens in Treatment

Good news: In general, doing anything is better than doing nothing. However, some treatments work better than others. For this chapter, I want to demystify what happens when a patient with purging disorder starts treatment. Using evidence from case studies (my own and those of others) and from controlled treatment trials, I describe what kind of help is most useful. I share what the treatments entail in some detail to help patients and clinicians recognize whether their treatment approach is supported by research. I also note how much improvement these treatments produce (spoiler alert: It's not 100%). I then offer some thoughts on how to tailor treatments to enhance their success for patients with purging disorder. Finally, I've listed some treatment "do's and don'ts" at the end of the chapter.

TREATMENT TEAM APPROACH

No single medical or mental health specialty possesses the necessary expertise to address all the ways that purging disorder impacts a person's health. Effective treatment requires a team of health care professionals working together. Team members should include, at minimum, a physician, a dietitian, and a therapist. They should be licensed to practice in their respective areas and should respect the expertise of fellow team members. This ensures that all team members take responsibility for their own work with a patient while coordinating with other team members to avoid contradictions and redundancy of effort.

A physician covers a patient's physical health and safety. Chapter 6 detailed all the ways that purging disorder causes medical problems. A physician should integrate care specific to purging disorder with ongoing care appropriate to the patient's age and health status. For children and adolescents, a pediatrician should serve in this role. For adults, a general practitioner or primary care physician could serve in this role, or a physician in internal medicine may be appropriate. Results from the initial medical exam may indicate the need for a specialist, and the physician in charge of the patient's overall medical care should include that specialist in the team. Medical complications, interventions, and side effects need to be fully understood by all treatment team members to ensure compassionate care.

A dietitian guides healthy eating practices by adding expertise in the body's nutritional needs. Dietitians have training in dietary sources of nutrients and the association between nutrient intake, energy expenditure, and integrity of bodily systems, including regulation of fluids, temperature, and body weight. A dietitian is not the same thing as a nutritionist. Sadly, the names for these professions could not be more misleading. On the face of it, you would think that a dietitian would prescribe diets whereas a nutritionist would improve nutrition. However, in the United States, dietitians are licensed health professionals with the appropriate training to help eating disorder patients develop healthier eating patterns. In contrast, nutritionists have no specific training or licensing requirements. Most patients with purging disorder—in fact, most people with any access to media of any kind—have been flooded with misinformation on what they should eat and when. A dietitian is the appropriate professional to address questions of what nutrients a body needs to function within normal limits. Otherwise, these questions will emerge in psychotherapy with a therapist who doesn't have specific training or expertise in nutrition.

A therapist implements an intervention to achieve symptom remission, including both thoughts and behaviors that characterize purging disorder and their emotional and cognitive antecedents and consequences. Therapists often help patients with interpersonal difficulties and challenges related to life transitions that impact purging disorder symptoms. Therapists can come from a range of professional disciplines, including psychiatry, clinical psychology, counseling psychology, and clinical social work. Beyond their potential role as a therapist, psychiatrists may be members of the treatment team to provide medication. There are no FDA-approved medications for the treatment of purging disorder. Medication may be prescribed to treat co-occurring disorders, including depression or anxiety disorders. When using any medication in purging disorder, it's important that patients take the medication at a time when they will not induce vomiting and to refrain from laxative use. Otherwise, therapeutic doses may not be achieved.

The Additional Resources section provides information that may help identify established treatment teams with experience in eating disorders. Alternatively, patients can create their own treatment team from professionals near them. The Additional Resources section also lists ways for health professionals to gain additional information and training. In forming a team, it's important to find individuals who will communicate effectively with one another. This requires respect for expertise beyond the health professional's own area and trust in other professionals.

When I was working at Massachusetts General Hospital's eating disorders program, a group of us brought our lunches to a conference room every Friday for a team meeting. Our group included psychologists, psychiatrists, dietitians, physicians, and trainees. I found our weekly meetings to be incredibly valuable to my own work. Knowing that a dietitian was already talking to my patient about a food plan protected me from getting drawn into a conversation about what she should eat. This was important because the specific content of her diet extended well beyond my expertise. Instead of getting bogged down in details about the relative merits of whole grain bread over oatmeal, I could support my patient's work with her dietitian by addressing my patient's anxiety about eating carbohydrates. It's appropriate for a dietitian to talk about how many vitamins are fat soluble or to discuss whether a vitamin deficiency can be addressed by adding more fat to a patient's diet. And then it's appropriate for the therapist to discuss a patient's emotional reaction to consuming fat. Communication among treatment members can also protect a dietitian from inadvertently reinforcing black-and-white thinking about food while extolling the virtues of whole grains over simple carbohydrates. Whole grain bread may have many advantages over a donut, but donuts are part of the real world. Patients benefit from learning how to eat a donut without feeling horrible about themselves. A team-based approach with strong communication helps keep everyone on the same page in supporting positive change for their patient, and it becomes a wonderful support network for professionals working with eating disorder patients.

PSYCHOEDUCATION

Many treatments begin with some form of psychoeducation. Psychoeducation should provide a lot of information to patients about their purging disorder, what maintains the disorder, and why a chosen treatment facilitates recovery. The content of psychoeducation will depend on the clinician's training. Both individuals with purging disorder and clinicians treating purging disorder represent important audiences for this book because the *whole book* contains information that could be used during psychoeducation. The following section may be especially helpful and is directed toward both clinicians and patients, but everyone is welcome to read it!

When done well, psychoeducation reinforces a lot of the costs of not changing, potential for change, and the rewards of changing to enhance motivation for treatment. For example, most patients identify damage to their bodies as a cost of purging. Clinicians can reinforce the high price of purging by laying out the specific medical consequences of purging during psychoeducation and reviewing findings from a patient's medical evaluation. Most patients also identify weight gain as a cost of not purging. In psychoeducation, clinicians can share that purging largely eliminates water from the body and, by itself, is an ineffective means of weight control. Researchers at the University of Pittsburgh conducted a study in which they had patients binge and purge within a private research suite so that they could collect vomit and compare its nutritional composition to food consumed. About two-thirds of the calories consumed were not expelled by vomiting. And the amount retained was not proportional to the amount consumed. About 1,000 calories were retained after vomiting, regardless of how much patients ate, suggesting that, in purging disorder, most of what's eaten before vomiting won't come back up. Importantly, this study was conducted in patients with bulimia who were bingeing on large amounts of food, and it's unknown whether the same results would be found in those with purging disorder. However, many of the basic mechanics of digestion work against self-induced vomiting as an effective means of weight control. Our bodies are designed to digest food the second it hits our mouths, with sugars being dissolved by saliva and directly absorbed into our bloodstream through the membranes in our mouths. In a liquefied state, food moves from the stomach to the intestines within minutes. Remember, we see peak gut hormone responses to food within 15 minutes! Laxatives move solid waste through the intestinal tract at a faster rate and decrease the opportunity for nutrients to be absorbed through the small intestine into the bloodstream. However, the body reacts by releasing chemicals that counteract these effects, such that more laxatives are needed to produce the same effects. Similarly, diuretics increase urination, which eliminates water from the body, but diuretic abuse contributes to the body releasing chemicals that cause water retention. Although purging may seem to work initially, patients eventually find themselves in an arms race with their own biology. For these reasons, by itself, purging locks patients into a cycle of harming their bodies without affecting their weight beyond the effects of chronic dehydration. When patients discontinue laxative use, it's important for them to consume plenty of water, stay physically active, and consume a diet with fresh fruits and non-starchy vegetables and whole grains. Similarly, when patients discontinue diuretic use, they should drink plenty of water. Given that they may already be suffering from bloating and swelling, it may be difficult for them to believe that more water is the answer. However, water will help their kidneys flush out the excessive factors their bodies released to counteract the effects of dehydration. Fortunately, it doesn't take long for the body to adjust and get back to normal, and psychoeducation prepares patients for initial discomfort and teaches them healthy approaches to support normalization of bodily functions.

For patients who experience a loss of control over their eating, psychoeducation explains the link between dietary restriction and loss of control. Substantial research supports that when we try very hard to refrain from a thought or action, we often do the exact thing we're trying to avoid. Try not to think about a white bear, and you think about a white bear. Try not to eat a chocolate chip cookie, and you eat a chocolate chip cookie. Part of this may reflect the attention required to not eat—refraining from food requires effort, and that requires attention. However, paying that much attention to food increases the power it has over your every waking thought. In addition, as we discussed in chapter 5, the longer we go without eating, the higher our ghrelin levels get and the stronger the signal to the brain that we must eat. If a patient wants to stop feeling a loss of control over eating three cookies, there are really only two logical options. Option 1: Never eat three cookies. Option 2: Accept that eating three cookies is perfectly okay. Between these two options, the second one has a much greater likelihood of succeeding over the long run. Thus, the key to not losing control over eating is to stop restricting food intake and to respond to internal cues of hunger and fullness as a guide.

Although psychoeducation would typically be a part of treatment after a course of treatment has been selected, psychoeducation also may be used during assessment to describe the psychotherapy options available for purging disorder. Initial considerations include a patient's age and motivation, the scope of problems to be addressed in therapy, and evidence that a given treatment works for those problems. However, once treatment is initiated, it's useful for clinicians to remain mindful of the pros and cons of different treatment options in relation to the specifics of a patient's case.

PSYCHOTHERAPY FOR PURGING DISORDER: WHAT ARE THE OPTIONS?

Although all sorts of treatments have probably been tried with purging disorder, like Las Vegas, what happens in therapists' offices stays in therapists' offices. And there hasn't been a lot of published work on the treatment of purging disorder. In particular, at the time of writing this chapter, there are *no* randomized controlled treatment trials (RCTs) specifically focused on patients with purging disorder. An RCT is a specific type of study in which patients are randomly assigned to an active treatment group or a control group. The control group might receive no treatment and only complete the same assessments completed by those receiving active treatment (assessment-only control), or the control group might receive an alternative treatment (active control group). By randomly assigning patients to be in either the treatment or the control group, each group represents a random sample of the patients who might receive the treatment being studied or might not. Over time, without any treatment, some people would get better on their own. By comparing people in each group over time, we can see whether the improvements in the treatment group were superior to those in the control group. Beyond natural changes over time, the act of receiving treatment is enough to promote recovery for some individuals even if the treatment itself isn't particularly powerful or effective. When comparing two active treatment conditions, we can see whether one treatment produced better outcomes than another. Because they produce very informative results, RCTs are considered the gold standard of evidence for a treatment, and comparison between an active treatment group and an active control group is considered the strongest level of evidence for identifying a superior treatment (Figure 8.1).

The absence of any RCTs focused on purging disorder represents a critical gap in research. This gap means that we have to rely on a combination of case studies, case series, and RCTs that have included cases of purging disorder among other eating disorders. Patients with purging disorder have been included in RCTs of three kinds of therapy: family-based treatment in adolescents, cognitive-behavioral therapy (CBT) in adolescents and adults, and integrated cognitive affective therapy (ICAT) in adults. Of these, CBT has been studied the most in eating disorder samples that include patients with purging disorder, whereas family-based treatment has the most support across a range of eating disorders in children and adolescents. There is an excellent case study detailing the use of CBT in an adolescent with purging disorder following an attempt to use family-based

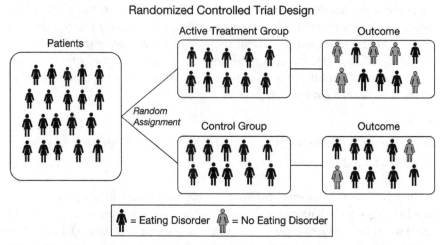

Figure 8.1 Design of a randomized controlled trial to determine treatment efficacy.

treatment. Thus, I'm going to start with descriptions of family-based treatment and will then discuss CBT.

In the interest of transparency, my own doctoral training emphasized the use of CBT as an evidence-based treatment for a range of mental disorders, and I personally have more training and experience in the use of CBT than in any other intervention. For example, the dialectical behavior therapy I mentioned in the previous chapter is a form of CBT. In addition, I have provided training and clinical supervision in the use of CBT to doctoral students in clinical psychology. However, this chapter is not intended to provide treatment or training. A single chapter is insufficient for either of these goals. Instead, the chapter is intended to describe family-based treatment, CBT, and ICAT to help both patients and clinicians recognize key components of each treatment. This can guide patients' efforts to find treatment providers and clinicians' efforts to find training. The Additional Resources section includes information to support both endeavors.

CASE STUDY FOR TREATMENT OF AN ADOLESCENT WITH PURGING DISORDER

Clinical psychologist Dr. Robyn Sysko worked with a 16-year-old girl, "Kaitlin," seeking treatment for purging disorder at the Columbia Center for Eating Disorders in New York. Kaitlin's BMI placed her in the 19th percentile, meaning that she was thin compared to her peers but not underweight. Reflecting the extent to which purging disorder is *not* a subthreshold eating disorder, Kaitlin vomited approximately five times per day. She purged in response to feeling a loss of control over her eating when she deviated from her planned diet—but the deviations weren't large. She also purged in response to generally feeling "out of control" in her life or when she felt emotional distress. At the time Kaitlin started treatment, one published RCT had demonstrated that family-based treatment was superior to individual therapy in adolescents with bulimia and purging disorder: After 6 months of treatment, 4 out of 10 patients in family-based treatment were symptom free compared to only 2 out of 10 patients in supportive psychotherapy. Because Kaitlin was a teenager living with both parents who were motivated to help her recover, Dr. Sysko initiated family-based treatment.

In family-based treatment for adolescents, the patient's family members are part of the treatment team. Following the intake assessment, the first session focuses on raising awareness and anxiety in parents and putting them in charge of regulating their child's eating. Parents are supported in developing methods to get their child to eat without restricting and without purging. Unlike prior incarnations of family therapy, family-based treatment does not blame the parents for their child's eating disorder. Instead, treatment empowers parents to implement changes at home to support recovery, similar to how nursing staff would encourage patients to eat during inpatient or residential treatment. In this example, we can see that a nurse doesn't have to be blamed for why a patient wasn't eating before to help them start eating now. This exact same model can be applied to parents. Family-based treatment has three phases: (1) refeeding the patient, (2) negotiations for a new pattern of relationships, and (3) termination. The first phase encourages parents to develop their own strategies for feeding their child and preventing purging. Once patients show willingness to eat without purging, the second phase focuses on other family issues that impact the child's symptoms and the parents' ability to support healthy eating. After patients have stopped purging and are free of other weight control behaviors (restricting food intake, excessive exercise), the focus shifts to encouraging a healthy relationship between the child and parents. This is important because any eating disorder represents a crisis, making it a focus of interactions in families. Recovery from an eating disorder requires rebuilding relationships to support a child's development. In addition to the one RCT that had included patients with purging disorder among those with bulimia, several RCTs have supported the superiority of family-based treatment for adolescents with anorexia.

Kaitlin's first session of family-based treatment did not go well. Her parents viewed some of her eating disorder symptoms as healthy. Her father suggested working with a personal trainer and nutritionist to achieve a more consistent approach to "get healthy," and her mother suggested that if Kaitlin could lose "a few pounds," she would feel better and stop purging. Moreover, after arguments over symptoms and unrelated topics persisted throughout the first session, both Kaitlin and her father refused to participate in family-based treatment together. Prior research indicated that family-based treatment was less effective in families characterized by higher levels of critical comments, hostility, and emotional overinvolvement. For anorexia, family-based treatment has been successfully adapted to hold sessions with adolescents and parents separately when family conflict precludes joint sessions.

Based on their high level of conflict, Kaitlin and her parents agreed to continue family-based treatment separately. This continued for three additional sessions. However, over the course of these sessions, Kaitlin's vomiting increased to six to eight times per day, and she attributed this to increased conflict with her parents over her eating disorder. Another RCT that included patients with purging disorder among adults with a broad range of eating disorders. This study showed that CBT enhanced to apply broadly across different eating disorders was superior to an assessment-only control. At the end of treatment, over a third of patients receiving enhanced CBT had stopped purging compared to 3% of patients completing assessments over that time. Based on a poor initial response to family-based treatment and at least some support for CBT, Dr. Sysko suggested they change treatment to enhanced CBT in which she and Kaitlin would work together to eliminate her disorder. Although family-based treatment did not help Kaitlin, it remains an important option to consider for purging disorder, particularly for the treatment of younger children.

CBT seeks to alter the thoughts (also known as cognitions) and behaviors that form an eating disorder. The main body of the treatment addresses concerns about shape and weight as the core feature that drives the eating disorder, addresses extreme dietary restraint through prescription of a regular pattern of eating, and improves skills in managing the events and shifts in mood that often trigger eating disorder behavior. Enhanced CBT lasts for 20 to 40 sessions and is broken down into four phases. The first phase typically lasts four weeks with sessions twice a week to support rapid improvements early in treatment. During the second and third phases, sessions occur once per week. During the fourth phase, sessions are spaced out to once every two weeks and finally tapered to a final, one-month check-in session to encourage maintenance of improvements. Additional sessions can be added at any phase to ensure that patients achieve the aims of each phase before moving on to the next phase.

Following this format, Kaitlin initiated CBT's first phase with self-monitoring via a daily food diary. Every day, Kaitlin was asked to record what she was eating as soon after eating as possible and the context of food intake (time, setting, events surrounding eating, whether she felt a loss of control). In the same daily diary, Kaitlin was asked to record every purging episode as soon after it happened as possible and the context of purging (time, setting, events surrounding purging). In addition to having purging disorder, Kaitlin was also diagnosed with attention-deficit/hyperactivity disorder and struggled to remember to write things down as they were happening. Dr. Sysko and Kaitlin worked together to use her phone to remind her to complete her records. Every time Kaitlin checked her phone, a phrase would appear as a reminder to complete her diary. In addition, Dr. Sysko initiated between-session phone check-ins to solve problems related to self-monitoring. Phone check-ins occurred daily for the first week when in-person sessions were occurring twice per week and then gradually decreased and transitioned to Kaitlin calling Dr. Sysko to confirm she was self-monitoring. Dr. Sysko recruited Kaitlin's mother to develop a reward system with Kaitlin to receive small rewards (e.g., money to go to the movies) for completing her records.

Engaging in therapy is effortful, and the rewards of recovery don't happen overnight. Small rewards for completing each step along the path of positive change are completely appropriate at any age to reinforce progress. It's important to use small rewards to avoid confusion over why you're making the change (you're making the change to recover, not to get a trip to Hawaii). Otherwise, the change may not be maintained in the absence of the reward. It's also important to choose rewards that won't trigger eating disorder symptoms (e.g., going to the movies may be a safer option than buying clothes or going out for ice cream).

During self-monitoring, Dr. Sysko prescribed a regular pattern of eating, consisting of three planned meals and two snacks per day with no more than four hours between meals/snacks. This part of CBT was designed specifically to prevent binge-eating episodes in bulimia, which may be triggered by the physiological consequences of dietary restriction. As we saw in chapter 5, our bodies are ready to eat as soon as two hours after our last meal. Going too long between eating increases biological drives to eat that can leave you feeling like you might lose control. In purging disorder, we saw higher ghrelin levels. In addition to increasing the release of that hunger hormone, dietary restriction sets patients up to regard normal food intake as wrong because they're "supposed to" eat less. The prescription of a normal pattern of eating helps normalize the biological drive to eat and change harmful attitudes about food intake. Eating something for breakfast, lunch, a mid-afternoon snack, dinner, and an evening snack is reframed as a treatment success rather than a dietary failure.

Although Kaitlin was able to follow this plan on weekends, she struggled on school days because her friends skipped lunch. To address this, Kaitlyn engaged in a behavioral experiment of eating lunch with a single friend on the weekend to see how her friend would actually respond. The friend was completely fine with this. Although the idea that a person would be cool with a friend eating lunch may not seem groundbreaking, there's an important difference between thinking that something would probably be fine and experiencing that it was fine. The great thing about behavioral experiments is that they replace hypotheticals ("if I do this, then that will happen") with real-world experiences. Although real-world experiences aren't all unicorns and rainbows, they rarely involve the catastrophic outcomes predicted by someone struggling with an eating disorder. The success of this experiment allowed Kaitlyn to experiment with eating lunch with her friends at school and to experiment with eating foods that had previously been forbidden to determine whether the feared consequences would occur. They didn't.

Although self-monitoring reduced the frequency of Kaitlin's purging episodes, it didn't eliminate them. Self-monitoring increases people's awareness of their own behaviors, and many initially put forth more effort to improve. However, this benefit tends to go away because people habituate to monitoring. Habituation means that people go back to doing whatever they would have done without monitoring. If you've ever watched a reality TV show and wondered how someone could allow themselves to get into a screaming match on national TV, habituation is your answer (well, that, and exceptional casting). This means that self-monitoring alone is an insufficient treatment. To produce lasting change in vomiting, Dr. Sysko worked with Kaitlin to identify triggers for vomiting from her daily diaries. In looking at the context of purging, they could see what events preceded purging and what happened after. Kaitlin's triggers included eating forbidden foods, feeling excessively full or fat after eating, distressing emotions, disrupted sleep, and conflict with family or friends. All of these represented stressors, and purging was Kaitlin's attempt to cope.

Dr. Sysko introduced the goal of delaying the use of purging to cope with stressors. Rewards were earned for achieving longer and longer intervals between a stressor and purging and for using an alternative means to cope with stressors. In Kaitlin's case, this was listening to a favorite song. Alternative coping strategies include any activity that helps patients manage distress without harming themselves or others. It could be taking a walk, talking to a friend, playing with a pet, taking a hot bath, or going to the movies. The best kinds of coping strategies are ones that reduce distress and are fundamentally incompatible with the behavior you're trying to prevent. So, of the examples given, taking a hot bath is fine, but the fact that it involves getting naked and that the tub is right next to the toilet might make it less helpful. Taking a walk or talking to a friend offer the same stress-relieving benefit and are both completely incompatible with purging. Kaitlin's goal was to reach an hour between the stressor and purging. This represents a concrete, achievable goal and provides an opportunity for effects of stressors to subside on their own, to allow alternative coping methods to work, and to reduce the contents of the stomach through normal digestion.

Consistent with CBT designed for bulimia, Dr. Sysko weighed Kaitlin once per week during treatment. The goal is to prevent avoidance of information about weight while also preventing compulsive checking and reassurance seeking. In using CBT for bulimia, psychoeducation presents evidence that patients generally don't gain weight during treatment because as they reduce their dietary restriction, they will binge less, and the purging wasn't effectively eliminating all of the food consumed during binges. CBT for bulimia emphasizes the calories consumed during a binge. That's *not* relevant for purging disorder. Understandably, for Kaitlin, "this information did little to reduce Kaitlin's anxiety about weight gain."[1] Even though CBT dictates that patients should actively participate in their own weighing, Dr. Sysko adjusted this because psychoeducation wasn't sufficient to reduce Kaitlin's anxiety. Initially, Kaitlin got on the scale without looking at her weight but remained on the scale until her anxiety subsided. Over subsequent sessions, Kaitlin experienced reduced anxiety during weighing and was able to fully participate in weekly weighings and see her weight.

This kind of gradual exposure to an anxiety-provoking experience is central to many forms of CBT. The idea is to start with exposure to something that elicits anxiety but is not overwhelming and to remain in that experience until the anxiety subsides on its own. As part of a fight-or-flight response, anxiety will increase in the presence of a threat and then go down on its own. With repeated exposures, patients learn from their own experience that nothing bad happens just because they stepped on a scale (or just because they ate a cookie). This decreases anxiety in the future and makes it possible to meet the next anxiety-provoking challenge that had been previously avoided. Over the first four weeks of treatment with CBT, Kaitlin's purging decreased from eight times per day to two times per day.

I've just described in a fair degree of detail the first phase of CBT for Kaitlin. If you're using CBT as a patient or clinician, these should look familiar. The daily diaries are tedious, and weekly weighings are anxiety provoking. And just to provide some insight, no therapist enjoys subjecting patients to tasks that are boring or distressing. However, those daily diaries and weekly weighings are part of the ongoing assessment needed to understand what maintains the eating disorder symptoms and to determine whether targeting those factors is having any effect on symptom levels. If these aren't happening as part of therapy, then therapy is missing important components of CBT for an eating disorder.

The second phase of Kaitlin's treatment identified both mood swings and interpersonal conflict as maintaining factors for purging, and the third phase addressed these issues. These interventions are modeled on those used across a broad range of illnesses characterized by mood intolerance and interpersonal problems. The original case report provides additional information on how the second and third phases were implemented with Kaitlin, and most licensed therapists have considerable training and experience in these interventions. By the end of the third phase, Kaitlin was no longer purging and no longer experiencing loss of control over her eating. She continued to experience herself as fat but decided not to let that thought guide her actions.

The final phase of treatment transitioned from weekly sessions to sessions occurring every other week. At this point, Kaitlin took charge of developing her own goals and identifying strategies to achieve them. This shift supports maintenance of treatment gains as patients take over the role of being their own therapist. Patients use skills developed during CBT to address new problems as they emerge in their lives. Anecdotally, patients completing CBT may share stories of extending what they've learned to help friends, family, and, occasionally, strangers. This final phase of Kaitlin's treatment also focused on relapse prevention, including how to distinguish between a momentary lapse versus when additional treatment is needed. Using skills learned in CBT to prevent a lapse from recurring is key to preventing relapse—which literally translates to "lapse again." In total, Kaitlin's CBT lasted for 29 sessions delivered over 36 weeks, reflecting approximately nine months. This represents a midpoint between a 20-session course over six months and a 40-session course over 12 months.

CBT is meant to be a time-limited treatment that focuses on the here and now rather than a multi-year exploration of personal development. However, it still requires a considerable commitment of time to complete. When I used the original CBT for bulimia in my therapy with Cara, the manual I was using indicated that the treatment was 20 sessions in length, which translated into eight sessions in the first four weeks, weekly sessions for the next nine weeks, and bimonthly sessions for the final six weeks, or four to six months total if additional sessions were needed. The original 1981 case series using CBT showed a duration of treatment just over six months, and nine of 11 patients had stopped bingeing and purging in the final month of treatment. My sense that my treatment with Cara wasn't working was based, in part, on unrealistic expectations for how quickly she would respond to treatment based on how the treatment worked for a group of patients with bulimia. I offer this observation to make two points. First, Cara didn't have bulimia. It was inappropriate to take findings from a group of patients with bulimia to set expectations for someone with purging disorder. Second, duration of treatment for *any* group of patients represents an average. Both clinicians and patients should be aware an average cannot represent each and every individual patient because of variability between patients.

Several RCTs have included patients with purging disorder among those with a range of eating disorders to evaluate CBT. In addition to the RCT showing CBT's superiority to assessment alone in adults with eating disorders, another RCT found that beginning CBT with an emphasis on early change produced better outcomes compared to starting with motivational interviewing before initiating CBT. Another RCT found no difference between family-based treatment and a version of CBT delivered through guided self-help to adolescents.

Guided self-help CBT is a more cost-effective option than treatments that rely completely on therapists for delivery. In the guided self-help version of CBT, therapists offered 10 weekly sessions with 3 monthly sessions and up to 2 sessions held with a close other, for a total of 13 to 15 sessions (vs. the 29 sessions received by Kaitlin or the original 20-ish sessions for CBT for bulimia). Therapists guide patients through a workbook that presents psychoeducation and exercises for patients to do on their own. Patients also receive support from a close other (similar to the support Kaitlin received from her mother). In the study comparing family-based treatment and guided self-help CBT, both treatments were expected to take six months. At the end of six months, less than a third of patients were free from vomiting. Twelve months after starting treatment, just over half of the patients were free from self-induced vomiting in both family-based treatment and guided self-help CBT.

A more recent RCT compared enhanced CBT to interpersonal therapy in adults with a broad range of eating disorders. CBT produced a greater reduction in vomiting, with almost half (46%) of patients no longer vomiting in CBT compared to just over a quarter (26%) in interpersonal therapy. However, at approximately one-year follow-up (two years after starting treatment), patients in both treatments were doing equally well. Over half (54%) had stopped vomiting. In prior research I've conducted on long-term outcomes in bulimia, I've interpreted similar patterns as showing that CBT speeds recovery but that patients receiving other treatments tend to catch up over time.

ICAT is the final form of treatment used for purging disorder that has been tested in an RCT. ICAT shares several features with enhanced CBT, including self-monitoring, meal planning, and strategies to cope with urges to engage in bulimic symptoms. Like enhanced CBT, it offers additional treatment for interpersonal problems and perfectionism if these are identified as factors maintaining eating disorder symptoms. Finally, it adds sessions on excessive self-control and self-neglect, as needed. Given similarities between ICAT and enhanced CBT, it's not surprising that no significant differences emerged in remission rates between these two treatments. At the end of treatment, over a third of patients in ICAT (37.5%) compared to under a fourth of patients in enhanced CBT (22.5%) were symptom free. It's not clear why enhanced CBT didn't produce as much recovery in this study as it did in prior studies. Changes reflected a 73% reduction in vomiting frequency in ICAT and a 76% reduction in vomiting frequency in enhanced CBT. These improvements were largely stable out to six-month follow-up.

Among the therapies that included patients with purging disorder in RCTs, enhanced CBT was specifically designed to be used across eating disorder diagnoses. And enhanced CBT has been tested in more RCTs with eating disorder samples that have included patients with purging disorder. In contrast, ICAT was originally developed as a new treatment for bulimia. And family-based treatment was adapted for bulimia from a treatment with initial support in adolescents with anorexia. For both the ICAT and family-based treatment RCTs, patients with purging disorder were included in an expanded definition of bulimia, not as patients with purging disorder. Thus, for adults and older adolescent patients, enhanced CBT represents a solid treatment choice, with both family-based treatment and ICAT as reasonable alternatives. Each of these treatments is designed to be tailored to the symptom configuration for a given patient. Each allows individualized conceptualization of underlying problems maintaining the illness beyond weight and shape concerns, such as interpersonal problems, emotion dysregulation, and perfectionism. Instruction on how to implement each of these treatments is beyond the scope of this chapter, but the Additional Resources section can guide therapists and patients to treatment manuals and workbooks for each intervention.

Although there have been no RCTs specifically focused on patients with purging disorder, RCTs that included patients with purging disorder didn't find any differences in treatment response between those with purging disorder and those with bulimia. Importantly, the absence of evidence should not be misinterpreted as evidence of absence. Specifically, RCTs haven't indicated how many patients with purging disorder were included. Based on what we saw in chapter 7, numbers were likely small—too small to adequately test for differences. Let me illustrate what I mean. Dr. Giorgio Tasca and colleagues working in the Regional Centre for Eating Disorders in Ottawa, Canada, described patients consecutively referred between 1996 and 2008. Among 1,422 female patients with confirmed eating disorder diagnoses and complete data, 415 had bulimia, 300 had anorexia, and 122 had purging disorder. Starting with these numbers, we can see that once again purging disorder is underrepresented in treatment-seeking groups compared to its presence in the general population. From these, about 3 out of every 10 patients with bulimia (126 women), almost 4 out of every 10 patients with anorexia (114 women), and about 2 out of every 10 patients with purging disorder (25 women) attended the day hospital program. With these numbers, we can see that even when patients seek treatment for purging disorder, they appear less likely to get treatment compared to patients with anorexia or bulimia. All patients received group CBT, and 48% of patients with purging disorder had a good outcome, defined as having a healthy BMI, no purging, and completing 11 weeks of treatment. Compared to outcomes from other studies, this sounds pretty good for only 11 weeks of treatment, and it supports the potential benefits of intensive treatment using CBT for purging disorder. However, this is less impressive compared to the 57% of patients with bulimia who achieved a good outcome and is somewhat more impressive than the 34% of patients with anorexia with a good outcome.[2] Although outcomes for purging disorder didn't show a statistically significant difference from those for bulimia, the outcomes are different enough to warrant concern about assuming that what works in bulimia works equally well in purging disorder.

Echoing this, Dr. Glenn Waller and colleagues evaluated CBT's effectiveness in 78 outpatients, including 4 patients with purging disorder, and noted "those with purging disorder showed a mixture of positive and negative outcomes, suggesting that this form of CBT is more suitable for those who binge-eat."[3] Only one of these four patients was free from an eating disorder after treatment, compared to over half of the other eating disorder patients. Based on these patterns, some adaptions may be warranted when applying CBT to purging disorder, similar to Dr. Sysko's approach in treating Kaitlin.

ADAPTING TREATMENTS FOR PURGING DISORDER

In the prior chapter, I described the importance of discussing potential weight gain frankly during motivational interviewing with purging disorder patients. This frank discussion may extend to adapting the psychoeducation piece of CBT on this topic. In CBT, patients are told that their weight is unlikely to change during treatment, and the weekly weighings are meant to reinforce that. If patients stop restricting their food intake, why don't they gain weight? Because patients who binge consume a lot of calories during binge episodes and purging doesn't get rid of those calories. For purging disorder, there are no large binge episodes, which means that there's no symptom driving increased calorie intake that a regular pattern of eating will prevent. Given that purging contributes to dehydration, weight gain may be more likely to occur in purging disorder. In Nicole Johns' discharge summary, her intake weight was 133 lbs. and her discharge weight was 140 lbs. A significant predictor of weight gain during treatment is the difference between a patient's highest prior weight and their weight when treatment begins. This should be used as a guide for the likelihood that patients may gain weight during psychoeducation rather than suggesting that their weights won't change.

As described in chapter 5, individuals with purging disorder are likely to experience excessive fullness, nausea, and/or stomachache as triggers for self-induced vomiting, and this appears to be linked to their unique physiological response to food intake. Therapists should acknowledge this biologically based barrier to keeping food down when encouraging them to discontinue purging. Given the physical discomfort and anxiety associated with eating and that purging may represent an attempt to avoid or alleviate these feelings, in-session exposure and response prevention may be useful to work through these issues. An in-session meal is a component used in family-based treatment that could be adapted for these purposes.

I covered exposure when discussing how Dr. Sysko approached weighing Kaitlin on a weekly basis. In this example, being exposed to her weight was anxiety provoking and the response would be to step off the scale to make the anxiety go away. Having Kaitlin remain on the scale until her anxiety subsided represented response prevention. In the case of having a patient consume food during a therapy session, eating food exposes the patient to potential anxiety and increased stomach discomfort and the response would be to vomit to get rid of both. Having a patient eat and not vomit would represent exposure and response prevention. Indeed, this was the successful approach Dr. Tuckwell employed with his patients in the late 1800s. Therapists today can work with patients to develop a hierarchy of foods from easiest to hardest to keep down. The idea of creating a hierarchy was also reflected in the example of Kaitlin's weighings. Kaitlin didn't start with getting on the scale and looking at her weight. That would have been too anxiety provoking. If a patient starts with something that is too challenging, this can create a stronger anxiety response by reinforcing how awful the experience was. Instead, the exposure should elevate anxiety in the therapist's presence without being unmanageable. A therapist's presence can increase the amount of discomfort a patient finds manageable. If eating three cookies would feel like a loss of control and trigger overwhelming feelings of anxiety and stomach discomfort, then an exposure could start with two cookies or even one cookie. Across sessions, patients work up through their hierarchy, starting with exposures that are challenging but manageable and then progressing to exposures that are more challenging. Between sessions, patients practice exposure to eating and preventing a purging response on their own as homework. The series of exposures increases comfort with eating normal amounts of food across a variety of foods both in therapy and in their daily lives.

The greatest limitation of CBT for treating purging disorder is the absence of methods to directly address purging. In that original 1981 article, Dr. Christopher Fairburn had written, "Interestingly, it does not seem necessary to tackle the self-induced vomiting: this ceases once food intake is under control."[4] This will not be true for those who purge without experiencing a loss of control over eating. More critically, these individuals haven't even been included in any of the RCTs using enhanced CBT to treat eating disorders. Not all purging follows food intake, especially for those who use laxatives or diuretics, as neither requires the presence of food in the stomach. And you can't count on purging to just stop on its own. Similar to Dr. Sysko's work with Kaitlin, it's important to consider the emotional context of purging. As described in chapter 4, we found that women experienced significant increases in positive emotions over the course of the day on days they didn't purge compared to days they did. This finding may not be immediately apparent when reviewing the daily diary collected as part of enhanced CBT, because we typically ask, "What happened before you purged?" not "What didn't happen before you purged?" The answer to that second question may be as simple as feelings of happiness, confidence, and security. And there's an intervention to increase those feelings, behavioral activation.

Behavioral activation, an intervention originally used in depression, could provide a protective emotional environment against purging. This intervention identifies activities that bring a person happiness and then assigns those activities to be completed each day as homework, just like you would assign the daily food diary for homework. If a person used to enjoy going to the public library to read *Better Homes and Gardens*, then that would be an activity the person is assigned to complete. This is another form of behavioral experiment. People withdraw from activities they used to enjoy because they believe they can no longer enjoy them at all. This deprives them of a source of happiness through a self-fulfilling prophecy. Here the patient's experiment tests whether or not they still can enjoy the activity. Behavioral activation research indicates they can and will. Borrowing from the long-running Nike ad campaign, the key is to "Just do it."

In addition to providing an emotional environment to protect against purging, it's important to find better ways to cope with emotional distress. As we saw in Kaitlin's case, enhanced CBT incorporates a focus on emotional regulation skills that includes alternative coping responses to stress. However, this focus comes later in treatment. In adapting CBT for purging disorder, it may be important to improve emotion regulation skills earlier in treatment and add behavioral activation for those whose purging is not triggered by loss of control eating. Integrative modalities therapy for eating disorders is a newer treatment that takes approaches from a range of evidence-based treatments and offers greater flexibility in ordering treatment targets and interventions to achieve symptom improvement. One clear advantage that integrative modalities therapy offers comes from conceptualizing purging as an avoidance behavior rather than a compensatory behavior. This broader view of the function of purging includes using it to avoid weight gain from food intake as well as using it to avoid difficult emotions. At the time of this writing, there have been no RCTs of integrative modalities therapy. Similarly, there have been no RCTs examining any of the suggested adaptions for purging disorder because there have been no RCTs focused on purging disorder. This means that clinicians treating patients with purging disorder need to assess outcomes individually for the patient as treatment progresses and adjust as indicated, similar to the excellent approach modeled by Dr. Sysko in her case study.

GENERAL TIPS ON GETTING THE MOST OUT OF TREATMENT

Unfortunately, while it's true that doing almost anything is better than doing nothing, there are some instances in which well-intentioned treatments don't help as much as they could or might even do more harm than good. Because therapy involves both the patient and therapist, each person holds some responsibility for getting the most out of treatment, and I want to address each person with some general tips that might help. The following tips are directed first to patients and then to therapists; however, everyone's welcome to read them—these aren't secret tips.

To patients:

1. Do not strengthen the factors that maintain purging. Beware of interventions that direct you to restrict your food intake based on inferences about food allergies or food sensitivities as triggering gastric problems. Before using any of these, get tested. Given what we know about purging disorder, efforts to restrict food intake to "safe" foods in the absence of a true allergy are likely to reinforce unhealthy rules that increase the risk of purging when rules are broken. Similarly, beware of treatments that emphasize a goal weight to define eating as healthy. A lot of these are promoted through popular media, friends, or family. We saw in Kaitlin's case how her father thought a personal trainer would help her develop a "healthier" diet and how her mother thought that if she could just lose a little weight, she'd feel better about herself and stop purging. All of this reflects how culturally embedded eating pathology is in our society. Getting stuck on a goal weight contributes to overvaluation of weight or shape on self-evaluation, and this is a barrier to recovery.

2. Prioritize the therapist's approach over the therapist's experience. Although it might be tempting to conclude that anyone with decades of experience treating eating disorders must know everything there is to know about treatment, that's just not true. I can pretty much promise you that, right now, no therapist has that much experience treating purging disorder. I really hope that changes, and I really hope this book helps. But in the meantime, less experienced therapists can be very effective if they are up to date on the research literature, well trained on approaches that are likely to work, and open to consulting with other eating disorder professionals. A more experienced therapist using this approach will also be very effective. The only way to know what approach a therapist uses is to ask. What is the basis for their treatment recommendation? Are they using an evidence-based treatment? If so, which one? If they are using an evidence-based treatment, this means there are published guides for how to conduct the treatment (many of which you can locate through the Additional Resources section). Then compare what happens in therapy with what's supposed to happen in treatment.

3. Don't stick with a clinician you don't like. We're all human beings, and we can't like everyone all the time. If there's just something about your therapist that rubs you the wrong way, that will make it harder to trust them and try new things. It doesn't mean that there's anything wrong with either of you, just that there isn't a good fit between you. A therapeutic relationship is like any relationship, and it's okay to be selective.

4. On the other hand, don't stick with a clinician just because you like them. Liking your therapist is a prerequisite for working with them effectively. However, it's one of those "necessary but not sufficient" kinds of things. A therapist is not your friend. This is a person who

is professionally responsible for helping you get better. Forming a friendship with your therapist could actually work against making progress together. You may be less willing to disclose something if you think it might hurt your therapist's feelings or disappoint your therapist. You can't prioritize your therapist's feelings over sharing information crucial to ongoing assessment and treatment of your eating disorder. Unlike friendships, therapeutic relationships are supposed to be one-sided, and it's the patient who is supposed to gain from the work together. Although the therapist may experience professional fulfillment from helping others (I hope they do!), the patient isn't there to meet the therapist's needs for professional fulfillment, self-esteem, or anything else. That's why therapists get paid money. Even if you really, really like your therapist, if you're not improving and there's no clear plan to help you get better, you should work with someone else who could offer alternative treatment approaches.

5. Be open to change. The point of therapy is to recover from your eating disorder, which means changing thoughts, feelings, and behaviors. Making changes requires effort, and not all of the changes will feel good. In fact, many changes will provoke anxiety. You may feel tempted to debate or negotiate with your therapist to help them understand why you can't or couldn't do something. Instead, when facing a difficult change, remind yourself that all you're being asked to do is give something a try. That's the only way you'll find out if it works for you.

6. Advocate for your needs. Mental health professionals are not mind readers. The only way your therapist can know how you're doing is if you tell them. If you need something, let your therapist know. Then work together to develop a strategy to make sure your needs are met. For example, if it's stressful to ask for time off from work to attend sessions during working hours, is it possible to move your session to the early evening or to your lunch break? If you move your session to your lunch break, can you eat lunch during your session? Would you feel more comfortable sitting somewhere else during your sessions? Say something. Expressing your needs represents an act of trust, and getting your needs met will strengthen that trust. Giving your therapist the opportunity to build trust in your relationship will help you make positive changes in treatment.

To therapists (again, everyone else is welcome to read these also):

1. Reflect on the basis of your treatment recommendations. Clinical experience is valuable when it is integrated with published research findings. Unless your patient flow is incredible and your ability to track outcomes is superhuman, it's difficult to understand which prior experiences will or will not be relevant with a new patient. Findings from RCTs give you a huge head start on sorting this out.

2. Avoid a "one size fits all" approach. Even the best treatments don't work for everyone. If you look at the percentages who recover using any treatment, it isn't 100%. While RCTs are important for generating conclusions about what is most likely to be effective, findings from RCTs will not be true for every patient. If a patient is not responding to treatment or is getting worse, it's important to try something else. Dr. Sysko started Kaitlin with family-based treatment because it had stronger evidence from an RCT than CBT. And then she shifted to CBT when the first five sessions of family-based treatment yielded nothing but an increase in vomiting frequency. Your patient's response in treatment is another form of evidence that should be considered.

3. But don't give up on a treatment just because it's not working as fast as you hoped. Some patients will make rapid improvements during treatment, and those individuals tend to have the best outcomes. However, recovery follows a winding path and takes longer than improvement. If the frequency of purging has gone down, this is evidence that treatment is working even if a patient is still purging three months into treatment. Keep working at it. Have a plan for what each step will involve and the expected outcomes, and understand how each outcome prepares the patient for the next step forward. If the patient gets stuck or experiences a setback, both you and the patient should understand that these are expected. Determine whether the patient might need to go back to a previous step and work on getting that more firmly established or whether the current step can be broken down into smaller, more manageable parts. It may take a year (or more) to eliminate purging.

4. Seek ongoing training. Whatever treatment approach you learned during graduate and postdoctoral training will continue to evolve over time. Some refinements may not make a huge difference. Others will.

5. Seek consultation with other clinicians working with patients who have eating disorders. Whether this is your 1st or 51st patient with purging disorder, using another professional as a sounding board can help reveal certain assumptions or errors in implementation that could undermine treatment efficacy. It can help identify alternative approaches to a problem if you reach an impasse during treatment. Another set of eyes on your work will only make the work stronger.

6. Do not let fears drive your decisions. For example, out of fear of overwhelming a patient, you may be tempted to play it safe during an exposure. To work, an exposure must involve some anxiety. This means being okay with asking patients to try something they won't like. If you avoid an exposure exercise because it might provoke anxiety, why should patients risk an exposure for homework when they're alone? Similarly, you might be tempted to back off on some treatment requirements, like food diaries, because of how unpleasant they are for patients. Again, rather than avoiding a task because it's unpleasant, work with your

patient to figure out rewards for doing it. Life is filled with unpleasant yet important tasks. Finding palatable approaches to such tasks is a useful life skill.

7. Balance treatment fidelity with flexibility. One of the biggest misconceptions about manual-based treatment is that it reflects a one-size-fits-all approach and is ill suited to real-world settings. This isn't true. Every published RCT included real people as participants. As a researcher, I can promise you that participants aren't some special class of human beings. They forget appointments, don't follow instructions, and don't always tell the truth. Every struggle you encounter in practice has definitely occurred in the RCTs. Workshops are a great opportunity to learn from the people who developed and refined the treatments about the pitfalls they encountered and how they worked through them or what they would try next time. I started this chapter emphasizing the value of a team-based approach. This same value extends to teamwork between therapists and researchers, with each respecting the expertise of the other to enhance collaborative approaches to helping patients get better.

8. And, perhaps most importantly, assess treatment targets throughout treatment to see if what you're doing is helpful. We don't have nearly enough information on the best way to treat purging disorder. In place of RCTs to tell us what treatment works, your best option is to collect your own information by having your patient complete a symptom measure or recording information from daily diaries at *each* session. This information can be plotted on a graph. If a patient's symptoms are going down, this is evidence that you're delivering a treatment that works.

Outcomes Near and Far

What does the future hold for someone with purging disorder? When we first started asking this question, we could only look at the percentage of people (usually women) who reported that they ever had purging disorder and then how many currently had it to estimate likelihood of recovery. Based on this approach, the outlook was positive. The average length of illness was 10 months in cases identified in Italy, and 7 out of 10 women with a history of purging disorder (70%) were currently free of their illness. In Australia, nearly 9 out of 10 women (90%) were currently free of their illness. In addition to suggesting a very high likelihood of recovery, we couldn't know how deadly purging disorder was because we could only learn about it from people who survived and could tell us about their experiences. About 15 years have passed since purging disorder was first given a name, and new studies have followed the same people over time to directly measure who got better, who remained ill, and who died. Researchers have evaluated the impact of pregnancy on illness course and the impact of illness on pregnancy outcomes. And we're just beginning to scratch the surface of what factors increase the likelihood of recovery. This chapter describes what's been learned from these studies with the hope of providing a benchmark against which we can work as a society to improve purging disorder outcomes.

DEATH

Two studies have examined the likelihood of death in a group with purging disorder followed over time. The first study followed 219 inpatients for 9 years. They found 11 women had died, meaning that approximately 1 in 20 patients with purging disorder died within 9 years of hospitalization for their eating disorder. Intuitively, we know that 1 in 20 women is a high number. To determine whether purging disorder significantly increases the risk of death, we compare the number of deaths that occurred to the number of deaths expected based on these individuals' age, sex, and other demographic data. The ratio of observed deaths to expected deaths is called a standardized mortality ratio, and it revealed that patients with purging disorder were four times more likely to die than expected.

This represented a statistically significant increased risk of death for purging disorder patients. Researchers determined the cause of death for 7 of the 11 deceased patients. Five women died from medical complications from purging, including death due to renal failure, cardiac failure, and multi-organ failure, reinforcing the severity of the medical consequences of purging described in chapter 6. One woman died by suicide, reinforcing the link between purging disorder and suicide attempts described in chapter 7. Breast cancer caused the last death. Altogether, purging disorder contributed to 6 of the 7 deaths for which a cause could be determined.

Purging disorder patients were five times more likely to die by follow-up than were patients with bulimia, making purging disorder significantly more deadly than bulimia in this inpatient group. Given that all patients purged and required hospitalization, why would death be more likely in purging disorder? Two possible answers come to mind. First, purging disorder patients had suffered from their eating disorder for longer before getting treatment compared to those with bulimia or anorexia. Patients with anorexia and bulimia were about 25 to 26 years old when they were admitted and had been ill for almost 8 years. Patients with purging disorder were almost 29 years old and had been ill for almost 9 years at admission. In addition to being less likely to get treatment, those with purging disorder may wait longer to get treatment. This was especially true for patients who died. Patients with purging disorder who later died were almost 42 years old and had been ill for nearly 17 years when they were admitted to the hospital. This delay in getting treatment permits purging to do more damage to the body.

Second, medical complications from purging may be worse in those who only purge compared to those who binge and purge. In 164 pediatric eating disorder inpatients, those who only purged were more likely to be classified as having metabolic syndrome compared to those who binged and purged, those who only binged, and those with restricting eating disorders. Metabolic syndrome involves at least three of the following five risk factors for heart disease: high blood pressure, high blood sugar, high triglyceride level, low high-density lipid cholesterol level (the so-called good cholesterol), and a large waistline. And differences could not be explained by age or BMI. We already understand that purging is dangerous, and binge eating has been associated with its own set of medical complications. But it's also possible that binge eating represents a biologically driven defense that offers some protection against the ravages of purging. Returning to the comparison of those with purging disorder who died versus those who lived, the patients who lived were significantly more likely to have atypical binge episodes. These would be episodes where they felt a loss of control over their eating but didn't consume a large amount of food. Perhaps the act of giving in to the urge to eat represents a drive toward life. Perhaps the loss of control over eating caused distress and motivated them to get treatment sooner. Importantly, these data come from patients treated in an inpatient facility, likely representing the most severely ill patients among those with purging disorder.

The second study examined death as an outcome in 84 women with purging disorder drawn from the community and followed an average of 10 years after diagnosis. No deaths were found. In contrast to the inpatient sample, these women were an average of 24 years old and had been ill for less than 5 years when they were diagnosed. They were originally recruited to participate in one of three studies and were required to have BMIs that fell between 18.5 and 26.5 kg/m^2 to ensure that results reflected their eating disorder rather than consequences of being underweight or significantly overweight. The second two studies (each described in chapter 5) required participants to be free of any medical conditions that required medication. The third study also required them to be free of current depression, suicidal thoughts, and alcohol and drug use disorders. All of these requirements strengthened the conclusions we could draw from our biological studies and minimized potential risks of study participation. However, follow-up of these participants may not represent the true toll of purging because it excluded anyone who wasn't healthy enough to participate at baseline.

For me, the message is clear. Purging disorder can kill. Delaying treatment is dangerous. And, yet, so many people shared how long they silently suffered with purging disorder. One woman wrote, "I am a 45-year old woman who has been purging since I was 17 years old." Another woman wrote, "I have had it off and on for over 30 years, more on than off. [. . .] I have never told anyone about my purging disorder. No one knows but me and now you." And another woman wrote, "I've had it for 20 years. I have not told anyone of this yet, but it consumes me." These stories don't fit into a picture in which people recover in 10 months. What is the likelihood of recovering from purging disorder, and how long does it take?

RECOVERY

At least 11 studies have followed individuals with purging disorder to determine their outcomes anywhere from 11 weeks after they started treatment to 10 years after they were recruited from the community. Together, these studies collected information from 943 individuals with purging disorder who were alive at the time of follow-up (Figure 9.1). Approximately 2 out of 5 people (40%) no longer had an eating disorder at follow-up. About 1 in 5 still had purging disorder, whereas 2 in 5 had another eating disorder. For 1 out of 5, they had bulimia at follow-up, suggesting that purging disorder represented the first stage of an eating disorder that would later be characterized by large binge episodes and purging. For the remaining 1 out of 5, they still purged without bingeing, but less often than before, or they exercised compulsively without bingeing. If the definition of purging disorder expanded to include less-than-weekly purging or compulsive exercise as a purging method, then 2 out of 5 individuals (40%) would still have purging disorder at follow-up. The number with either anorexia or BED was so small across studies that it rounded to 0%.

We can break the studies down by duration of follow-up to get a sense of when recovery happens. For follow-up durations of less than one year, over 2 in 10 individuals have no eating disorder, and 3 in 10 still have purging disorder.

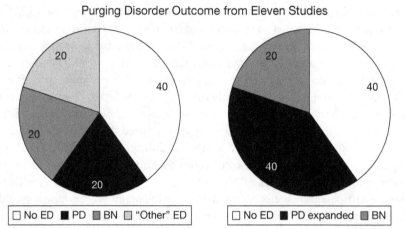

Figure 9.1 Outcome in purging disorder. ED = eating disorder; BN = bulimia nervosa; ED = eating disorder; PD = purging disorder.

For follow-up durations of at least one year but less than five years, 4 in 10 have no eating disorder, and just over 1 in 10 have purging disorder. For follow-up durations beyond five years, about 4 in 10 have no eating disorder, and over 2 in 10 have purging disorder. This suggests substantial improvement from one to five years as individuals have more time to recover from their illness. One study showed that the odds of recovery increased significantly over time. However, that likelihood stays stubbornly below 50% even as duration of follow-up extends to 10 years.

It also looks like people go from not having purging disorder to having it again as duration of follow-up increases beyond five years. One young woman described that she had been purging 3 to 5 times per week for the last 7 years and noted, "There have been months that I have gone without (silly, but I am trying to give my body a healing period), but I always come back." Another woman wrote, "Throughout the 10 plus years of dealing with this problem, I have had points where I have felt that I conquered the problem and points where it totally consumes my life." To capture patterns of improvement and relapse, you need to follow up with people repeatedly.

Three studies provided multiple follow-up assessments of individuals with purging disorder. One study provided data at the end of CBT treatment, at 6-month follow-up, and at 12-month follow-up in four patients with purging disorder. Two patients experienced decreased purging frequency after treatment, but it rebounded and doubled in frequency by 12-month follow-up. A study of 563 teens with purging disorder found that over a third got better and stayed better with a low likelihood of fluctuating back and forth. This study also found that nearly a third continued to have full or subthreshold purging disorder a year or more after diagnosis. The last study focused on a sample of pregnant women and provided particularly interesting findings on how pregnancy influenced symptom levels and vice versa.

PREGNANCY AND PURGING DISORDER

The Norwegian Mother and Child Cohort Study asked pregnant women about the presence of eating disorders during the 6 months prior to pregnancy, at 17 weeks of pregnancy, and again at 18 months and 36 months postpartum.[1] This means that the last assessment occurred when their children were three years old. Among the 92 women who reported purging disorder prior to their pregnancy, almost 8 out of 10 women (79%) reported no eating disorder at 17 weeks of pregnancy; the rest were evenly split between having purging disorder or another eating disorder. By 18 months after their babies were born, less than half (46%) were free from an eating disorder, meaning that approximately a third had relapsed. More than 1 in 10 women relapsed to purging disorder. By the time their children were three years old, over half of women (57%) reported no eating disorder, and about 1 in 10 had purging disorder. These data suggest that pregnancy represents a period in which purging is more likely to remit than to continue. Although there was some relapse after pregnancy, outcomes at three years look more promising than outcomes in other samples. Findings mirror Cara's experience with her pregnancy and purging disorder.

After I moved from Massachusetts to Iowa, Cara sent me a letter to let me know how she was doing. I was delighted to learn that she had recovered. After three years of working together, she was still purging when my fellowship at Massachusetts General Hospital ended. We discussed finding a therapist where she was currently working and living. She had been commuting over an hour each way to get to her weekly sessions with me after she had moved out of the Boston area. But she didn't want to work with another person. In her letter, she shared that she had a baby girl. Having a daughter committed her to being a good role model because she didn't want her daughter to ever struggle with the body image issues that had possessed her. She stopped purging and never started again. Both she and her daughter were healthy, and she expressed gratitude for our work together.

In addition to wanting to be a good role model once their children are born, many pregnant women discontinue their eating disorder during pregnancy because they want to protect their pregnancies. The Norwegian Mother and Child Cohort Study also examined the effects of purging disorder on women's health during pregnancy and their babies' health at delivery in a larger sample that included 292 women with purging disorder histories and over 40,000 women without eating disorders. Researchers examined high blood pressure during pregnancy (*preeclampsia*), gestational diabetes, delivery through cesarean section, breech presentation during delivery, slow progress during delivery, duration of pregnancy (*preterm birth*), the baby's birth weight, and the baby's Apgar score. The Apgar score measures the baby's color (appearance), heart rate (pulse), reflexes (grimace), muscle tone (activity), and breathing (respiration). Higher scores are better, and the test is administered at one minute and five minutes after birth. Across all measures, there were no significant differences between women with no history of eating disorders and those with a history of purging disorder.

Part of this good news likely reflects that most women who had purging disorder before they were pregnant may *not* have an eating disorder during their pregnancy. Part of this also may reflect that women who have never had an eating disorder experience nausea and vomiting during pregnancy. The researchers were very careful to ensure that women distinguished between vomiting deliberately to control their weight and vomiting due to morning sickness. In an earlier paper from the Norwegian Mother and Child Cohort Study, 70% of all pregnant women in the study experienced nausea, and 35% reported vomiting during their pregnancies. During the first four weeks of pregnancy, those with a history of purging disorder were over two times more likely to vomit compared to women without a history of an eating disorder, even though there were no differences in nausea. However, as their pregnancies progressed, those with purging disorder no longer looked significantly different from those with no eating disorder history on vomiting. Finally, although it appeared that women with a history of purging disorder were twice as likely to be hospitalized for excessive vomiting during pregnancy (*hyperemesis gravidarum*), the numbers were so small in both groups that they didn't differ significantly. This particular study only included 42 pregnant women with a history of purging disorder, and only one of these women was hospitalized for excessive vomiting. In a subsequent report including 292 women with histories of purging disorder, only two had excessive vomiting during pregnancy, and this did not differ from what was observed among women without eating disorders.

To the extent that vomiting is a well-recognized feature of some pregnancies, whatever risks it brings may not dramatically differ between those with and without purging disorder. This could mean that vomiting does produce negative outcomes, but the physical consequences may not depend heavily on the motivation behind the behavior. As such, these negative consequences may occur in both those with and without an eating disorder so that we see no differences between groups. Alternatively, it could mean that pregnancies are robust against the possible harms of vomiting unless it's severe enough to cause dehydration and weight loss. But this serious complication didn't differ between those with and without purging disorder in this study.

Now that I've offered this good news, I need to temper it with findings from an even larger study comparing pregnancy and neonatal outcomes between 7,542 women with eating disorders and 1,225,321 women without eating disorders in Sweden. Women with eating disorders were diagnosed with anorexia, bulimia, or an eating disorder not otherwise specified (EDNOS)—this last group would have included women with purging disorder along with a range of other disorders that didn't quite meet criteria for anorexia or bulimia. Key findings included that women with any eating disorder, regardless of diagnosis, were two times more likely to experience excessive vomiting (*hyperemesis*) during pregnancy and were more likely to have preterm births and deliver babies with smaller heads (*microcephaly*). In addition, both women with anorexia and those with EDNOS were twice as likely to experience low blood iron levels (*anemia*) during pregnancy. While none of these outcomes was specifically linked to purging disorder, their presence across eating disorder diagnoses is cause for concern and supports increased medical attention for patients with current or past eating disorders during pregnancy and delivery.

PREDICTORS OF OUTCOME IN PURGING DISORDER: WHO GETS BETTER?

Only three studies examined whether anything measured at baseline predicted who was most likely to recover at follow-up. One study suggested that a younger age at admission, fewer symptoms of depression, and fewer physical symptoms increased the likelihood of remission. A second study found that lower scores on measures of worry about the self, combined with higher scores on measures of harm avoidance, persistence, and self-directedness increased the likelihood of remission from purging disorder. Finally, a third study found that lower weight and shape concerns increased likelihood of remission. Aside from younger age and fewer physical symptoms, these predictors represent psychological factors related to mood, confidence, and body image. One question is whether these predictors can be modified by treatment to increase the chances of recovery for more people.

All three studies examined symptom frequency as a potential predictor of outcome, and none found an association. This suggests that an individual purging once a week and an individual purging multiple times per day do not clearly differ in their likelihood of remission. All three studies also examined duration of illness at baseline as a predictor of remission from purging disorder and found no association. This is unusual. Duration of illness is one of the more reliable predictors of eating disorder outcome for anorexia and bulimia. The longer someone has been ill at baseline, the longer they remain ill during follow-up. Although neither purging frequency nor duration of illness appears to predict the likelihood of remission in purging disorder, they may still be linked to the likelihood of medical complications and risk of death. Other nonsignificant predictors included age of illness onset, BMI, motivation to change, duration of inpatient treatment, relationship status, educational attainment, and total scores on general measures of psychopathology and eating pathology. This leaves us with only a few scattered clues as to why some people get better and others do not.

CONFLICTING OUTCOMES AND THE NEED FOR MORE RESEARCH

The two studies examining death in purging disorder provide very mixed findings. One study found no deaths, but it focused on a relatively young and healthy sample of women with purging disorder. The other study found that 1 in 20 patients had died at follow-up. However, this may reflect the worst possible outcomes for purging disorder because the group was drawn from patients requiring hospitalization for their eating disorder—so they were very ill. We also just don't know if there were deaths in the other follow-up studies. If we add the 11 reported deaths as outcomes to the 943 living individuals for whom follow-up data have been collected, this becomes 11 deaths out of 953 people, or a mortality rate of 1% instead of 5%. However, I don't think we can be quite that optimistic. Studies that rely on reaching people to get follow-up information can't distinguish among the reasons that people don't respond. Some never receive the invitation to participate because they've moved. Some don't respond because they don't want to participate. Some may be dead. My own view is that no one should die from purging disorder, making the six deaths known to be caused by purging disorder unacceptable.

Across all studies following those with purging disorder, most people don't continue to have purging disorder. In addition, considerable improvement continues to occur between the first and fifth year following diagnosis. Balancing this, studies suggest that most individuals with purging disorder continue to suffer with an eating disorder more than five years after diagnosis. Depending on how purging disorder is defined, the likelihood of remission and the likelihood of continuing to have purging disorder appear similar. Worse, an official diagnosis typically occurs several years after the onset of eating problems. This translates into too many people spending more than a decade of their lives purging. One woman wrote,

> I am a 51-year old woman who has suffered from this since 18 years of age. Continuously. I actually tried to calculate once the number of times I've purged over the years and the number was staggering! I have tried over the years to seek help but to no avail. I've always felt that I don't quite "fit in" with that of what is described as the "true" bulimic. So much so, that I've actually wished I had the willpower to be anorexic—just to receive such medical help.

We have to do better.

THE FUTURE OF PURGING DISORDER IN THE FIELD

Here I am at the end of the final chapter of this book, and I should be happy because I'm almost done. But I'm not satisfied by how the book is ending. I'm frustrated by the paucity of information for questions that we should have answered by now. And I'm wrestling with the feeling that we could be doing so much better as a field. Part of this feeling reflects my own standards, which tend to be high, and optimism, which tends to stray too far from reality. But part of this feeling reflects what I've seen my field accomplish. Bulimia nervosa was first named in 1979, officially included in the DSM-III in 1980, had a tailored psychotherapy in 1981, and has an FDA-approved medication for its treatment. This tells me that the field of eating disorders is capable of achieving an exceptional level of progress when we focus our efforts.

But it's hard to get the field to focus on an invisible problem. When I ask genetics researchers about purging disorder, I've been told, "It's so rare." When I ask treatment researchers about purging disorder, they tell me, "We don't see a lot of that in our program." But I don't think that purging disorder is that rare, and I think there's a different reason it's not showing up in treatment programs. You want a fun fact? Dr. Gerald Russell's seminal description of bulimia nervosa in 1979 was based on 30 patients seen over 6.5 *years*. After the DSM-III officially recognized bulimia, droves of patients who had been bingeing and purging poured into treatment. Whether they had been in treatment but misdiagnosed with anorexia or just hadn't thought they had a "real" problem, they were invisible to those responsible for studying and treating eating disorders before 1979. We get trapped in a cycle of studying what we define and then only recognizing what we study. I now see the same underrepresentation of purging disorder in treatment-seeking populations because it's an "other" eating disorder.

In the leadup to the DSM-5, I was invited to write two reviews on purging disorder and to present at a meeting for members of the DSM-5 Eating Disorders Workgroup. After the meeting ended, I had a candid exchange with the chair of the workgroup, Dr. Tim Walsh. I shared that I didn't think there was enough research on purging disorder for it to be included as an official eating disorder, on equal footing with anorexia and bulimia. It was 2008, and we didn't have any meaningful data on course, outcome, or treatment response. Having observed the avalanche of work accomplished on BED following its inclusion as a provisional disorder in the DSM-IV, I wanted the same thing for purging disorder in the DSM-5. That's not quite what I got. Purging disorder was officially named and included as an eating disorder, but it was folded into the broader category of "other specified feeding or eating disorder" along with four other named conditions.

Unbeknownst to me, the DSM-5 would unveil another condition that practically no one had studied, avoidant restrictive food intake disorder (ARFID). Based on its DSM-5 diagnostic code, it wasn't so much a new disorder as a reincarnation of the DSM-IV's feeding disorder of infancy or early childhood. But its new name (and acronym), new diagnostic criteria, and inclusion in a DSM-5 chapter of combined feeding and eating disorders led to an explosion of research on ARFID. Prior to the May 2013 publication of the DSM-5, a search of the online research database PubMed identified 20 papers on ARFID. Since May 2013, 138 additional papers have come out on ARFID. And now we have a CBT for ARFID, and you can order its treatment manual from major online booksellers.

After the DSM-5 came out, I asked a couple of members of the workgroup how something with so little evidence could be included in the DSM-5. I was told that it had to be included because so many kids were being brought into treatment because they were refusing to eat, and no one knew how to help them. I draw two conclusions from this. First, clinical researchers at university-based hospitals drive the major research initiatives in eating disorders. If they're not seeing a lot of patients with purging disorder, they're going to conclude that it's not that big of a priority. Second, my reservations about including purging disorder in the DSM-5 because we didn't know anything about how to treat it were clearly misguided.

The DSM-5 workgroup's deliberations were strictly confidential, so I'll never know whether purging disorder might have been included along with BED and

ARFID as an official eating disorder diagnosis. But I regret thinking of myself as a scientist who needed to be objective instead of as an advocate who needed to represent those suffering from purging disorder. Part of my hope in writing this book is that those with purging disorder will start advocating for themselves by seeking treatment and by refusing to be invisible to those in a position to help through clinical and research efforts.

Recently, I was invited to write a review on purging disorder for *Current Opinions in Psychiatry*. The invitation asked me to "help specialists remain up-to-date on research" by focusing only on recent publications. I found 13 studies that contributed to greater understanding of the prevalence, causes, and treatment of purging disorder published between January 2017 and May 2019. During this period, another eight articles included "purging disorder" as a keyword, but findings specific to purging disorder weren't reported due to insufficient sample sizes. Right now, what's getting published on purging disorder comes from a small number of very large-scale studies capable of yielding a sufficient number of individuals with purging disorder. But none of these studies set out to study purging disorder. At the time I'm writing this chapter, there are no federally funded studies of purging disorder in the United States.

Whenever purging disorder is included in research but there aren't enough cases to be examined separately, results for purging disorder are combined with those for "other" eating disorders or bulimia. This mirrors what's happened for purging disorder in RCTs. Blurring purging disorder with bulimia may become more common due to changes to the definition of binge eating in the most recent edition of the International Classification of Diseases (ICD-11) published in June 2018. In the prior edition, the ICD and DSM shared a single definition of binge eating. Now, the ICD-11 defines binge eating as "a distinct period of time during which the individual experiences a subjective loss of control over eating, eating notably *more or differently* than usual, and feels unable to stop eating *or limit the type or amount* of food eaten"[2] (emphasis added). The new definition of binge eating doesn't require a large amount of food and absorbs much, but not all, of purging disorder into a broader definition of bulimia.

I'm sympathetic with the rationale for this change. As one clinician wrote,

> I am a psychologist in private practice and very frustrated by the differential treatment of these patients [referring to patients with purging disorder] (relative to patients with AN [anorexia nervosa] or BN [bulimia nervosa]) by a major local insurer, in the context of recent parity law which covers AN and BN but not EDO NOS [eating disorder not otherwise specified]. My subjective experience has been that illness severity in some of the PD [purging disorder] patients I see is often equally severe and sometimes more severe than in some who meet criteria for AN or BN.

Under the ICD-11, many with purging disorder are eligible for better medical coverage because they meet full criteria for bulimia. Now, if someone with purging disorder is diagnosed with bulimia, they'll see a disorder that more closely matches their experiences in the ICD-11. Those are both good things. But there's a cost to this solution.

The new ICD-11 definition for bulimia differs from DSM-5 bulimia. We already know enough about differences between bulimia and purging disorder to know that ICD-11 bulimia will be a more heterogeneous group. This could impact the relevance of prior findings for bulimia, slow research advances for bulimia, and largely eliminate research advances for purging disorder.

Here is one example of how this could occur. Right now, fluoxetine (better known by its trade name, Prozac) is approved by the FDA to treat bulimia based on multiple double-blind, placebo-controlled randomized trials. In every single study establishing its efficacy, participants had large binge episodes. The effects of this antidepressant on bulimia appear to be independent of its effects on mood, and a much larger dose (60 mg) is required for bulimia than for depression (20 mg). Leading explanations for the mechanisms that make fluoxetine work focus on serotonin function and appetite regulation. The logic is that serotonin function is abnormally low in patients with bulimia (it is), serotonin is important to regulating appetite (it is), and fluoxetine improves serotonin function in patients with bulimia (it does). No part of this clearly applies to purging disorder. And no study has tested fluoxetine in purging disorder. So, what happens when physicians prescribe fluoxetine to patients with purging disorder because they can be diagnosed with ICD-11 bulimia? Based on several e-mails I've received, the results are disappointing at best. To me, this exemplifies the greatest cost of absorbing purging disorder into a broader definition of bulimia. This approach assumes there are no differences without ever fully testing whether this is true. Hopefully, the field will recognize that this change is premature.

We need studies designed to specifically examine purging disorder in a large enough number of people to increase understanding and improve interventions. The following wish list of studies could significantly advance progress on this problem:

1. Population-based studies of the prevalence and incidence of purging disorder in the United States and elsewhere. The two most recent nationally representative epidemiological studies of mental disorders in the United States were incapable of describing the number of people affected by purging disorder because of skip rules. It adds an average of only two minutes per interview to ask questions about purging and body image disturbance in everyone.

2. Network analyses of purging and purging disorder among social groups in large school and community-based samples to examine peer-based influences that could be leveraged in interventions to stem and even reverse the spread of purging.

3. More population-based twin and adoption studies of purging disorder to establish the contributions of genetic and environmental influences.

4. If twin and adoption studies support genetic influences to purging disorder, then molecular genetic studies can identify underlying

mechanisms contributing to purging disorder. In July 2019, *Nature Genetics* published an article documenting a specific set of genetic mutations in anorexia that influence metabolism based on DNA samples taken from 16,992 individuals with anorexia worldwide. Again, the field is capable of incredible progress, and purging disorder can be part of these efforts.

5. Neuroimaging studies of purging disorder to capture brain activity linked to the thoughts and feelings around purging, focusing on both emotional and physical sensations. Understanding what brain regions are involved in the unique experience of excessive fullness, nausea, and stomachache could identify new targets for treatment, particularly if we can link changes in brain activity to changes in symptom levels over time.

6. Open treatment trial of fluoxetine in purging disorder. Fluoxetine is effective in treating bulimia, obsessive-compulsive disorder, and depression, among other disorders. If it helps, then a randomized double-blind placebo-controlled trial of fluoxetine in purging disorder in a large sample could be conducted. If it doesn't, then alternative medications could be explored based on posited mechanisms for purging disorder.

7. Compare CBT adapted for purging disorder in an RCT to *any* of the following treatments: enhanced CBT, ICAT, family-based treatment or interpersonal therapy, again with a large enough sample of patients with purging disorder to adequately test which, if any, treatment is superior. This requires that people with purging disorder start seeking treatment and volunteer for treatment studies.

8. More longitudinal studies of purging disorder, including both short-term intensive ecological momentary assessment and long-term follow-up including repeated assessments to document maintenance factors, course, and outcome. To facilitate this, we need to agree on minimum thresholds for diagnosing purging disorder. The DSM-5 just stipulates "recurrent" purging without defining what this means. This may be the biggest difference between how the DSM-IV handled binge-eating disorder and how the DSM-5 handled purging disorder. We also need more long-term follow-up studies to examine vital status for *all* participants by matching records to national registries. Without this, not only is purging disorder invisible but its true cost to society remains invisible.

A big barrier to learning more about purging disorder is restricting ourselves to what we've studied in anorexia and bulimia. Without meaning to, this is another way of treating purging disorder as if it's just like anorexia or bulimia. When we find that factors relevant to anorexia or bulimia aren't relevant to purging disorder, this shows that purging disorder is different. But this approach doesn't yield new information on what is true and unique to purging disorder. So, the last item on my wish list is to ask questions about purging disorder that are more than just repeating what we've done for anorexia and bulimia. For my part, I'll keep working to understand why those with purging disorder feel compelled to eliminate normal or small amounts of food. I hope this work will produce novel insights that lead to innovative treatments.

We may not have any experts on the treatment of purging disorder, but we certainly have a lot of experts on what it's like to live with purging disorder. And I don't want to confuse my 20 years of studying purging disorder with the expertise developed from living with purging disorder every day. Every single item on my wish list requires individuals with purging disorder and eating disorder professionals to work together to improve outcomes for purging disorder through earlier identification, earlier treatment, commitment to evidence-based treatments, increased access to care, and greater understanding of what works in whom. This is a lot to ask, but we have shown an ability to accomplish a lot over a very short period of time. The key to our success is ensuring that we understand and accept the challenge before us.

NOTES

Introduction

1. The DSM has been colloquially referred to as the "Bible" of mental illness because of its profound impact in the field.
2. Because these were the first three women I saw, I planned to start treatment with all three. However, one did not return for therapy after her intake session, and another dropped out of treatment after her first three sessions. Cara worked with me for nearly three years, and my experiences with her impacted my understanding of purging disorder in ways that I am still discovering to this day.
3. Fairburn, C. G. (1985). Cognitive-behavioral treatment for bulimia. In D. M. Garner & P. E. Garfinkel (Eds.), *Handbook of psychotherapy for anorexia nervosa and bulimia* (pp. 160–192). Guilford Press, p. 171.
4. Ibid., p. 174.
5. Within a few weeks, we received hundreds of calls, including a call from the Cambridge Police Department informing us that we had 24 hours to remove all posters from telephone poles and other unauthorized locations or we would be fined $200 per poster. We got them down.
6. Within the field of eating disorders, we refer to these as "subjective binge episodes" or "subjective bulimic episodes" to capture the subjective experience of having eaten too much and to distinguish these from "objective binge episodes"/"objective bulimic episodes," in which individuals have eaten an amount of food that is definitely larger than most people would eat under similar circumstances. In all editions of the DSM, binge eating is defined as an objective binge episode, involving a large amount of food and a loss of control over eating.
7. American Psychiatric Association. (2013). *Diagnostic and statistical manual of mental disorders* (5th ed.). American Psychiatric Publishing (p. 353).
8. Johns, N. (2009). *Purge: Rehab diaries*. Seal Press (p. 11).
9. Ibid., p. 85.
10. Keel, P. K., Mitchell, J. E., Miller, K. B., Davis, T. L., & Crow, S. J. (1999). Long-term outcome of bulimia nervosa. *Archives of General Psychiatry, 56,* 63–69 (p. 64).

Chapter 1

1. Some might argue that there are four official eating disorder diagnoses in the DSM-5, anorexia, bulimia, BED, and avoidant/restrictive food intake disorder (ARFID). ARFID was included in the DSM-5 as a revision to the DSM-IV's feeding disorder

of infancy and early childhood. The definition of ARFID, its diagnostic code, and its placement immediately after pica and rumination disorder, which are feeding disorders in the DSM-5, suggest that ARFID is a feeding disorder, not an eating disorder. However, the distinction between feeding and eating disorders is not entirely clear or universally agreed upon.

2. Governor's Highway Safety Association (2019). Pedestrian Traffic Fatalities by State. https://www.ghsa.org/sites/default/files/2019-02/FINAL_Pedestrians19.pdf.

3. This phrase describes identifying biologically based differences to distinguish between two categories or classes. For example, in medicine, diabetes is divided into two types—type 1 and type 2. In type 1 diabetes, the pancreas no longer makes insulin and patients must take insulin through shots or a pump to survive. In type 2 diabetes, the pancreas continues to make insulin but the body is less responsive to that insulin, and the illness can often be managed through diet, exercise, and oral medication. Not producing any insulin and being resistant to the effects of insulin produce the same symptoms, but the differences in underlying biology and treatment justify separate diagnoses.

4. Russell, G. (1979). Bulimia nervosa: An ominous variant of anorexia nervosa. *Psychological Medicine, 9*, 429–448.

5. Within his own program of research, Dr. Stunkard was far more fascinated by night eating syndrome (NES). NES is another named and described condition included among the DSM-5 OSFEDs.

6. The DSM-IV Eating Disorders Workgroup included four psychiatrists and one clinical psychologist, of whom four were men and one (a psychiatrist) was a woman.

7. McCarthy, L. P., & Gerring, J. P. (1994). Revising psychiatry's charter document: DSM-IV. *Written Communication, 11*, 147–192 (p. 172). doi:10.1177/0741088394011002001

8. I'm glossing over a lot of rich detail available from the ethnographic study of the DSM-IV Eating Disorder Workgroup's process, included in McCarthy and Gerring (1994) referenced in the Source References section.

9. McCarthy & Gerring, p. 172.

10. Frances, A. (2012). DSM 5 is guide, not bible—Ignore its ten worst changes. *Psychology Today.* https://www.psychologytoday.com/blog/dsm5-in-distress/201212/dsm-5-is-guide-not-bible-ignore-its-ten-worst-changes.

11. McCarthy & Gerring, p. 172.

12. Ibid., p. 176.

13. https://icd.who.int/browse11/l-m/en#/http%3a%2f%2fid.who.int%2ficd%2fentity%2f509381842

14. American Psychiatric Association. (2013). *Diagnostic and statistical manual of mental disorders* (5th ed., p. 353). American Psychiatric Association.

CHAPTER 2

1. Bruch, H. (1978). *The golden cage*. Harvard University Press (p. vii).

2. It's not fully true for anorexia either.

3. Dwarfing the incidence of cervical cancer, which has 8.1 new cases per 100,000 females per year.

4. The one in Cambridge that almost cost us thousands of dollars in fines due to improper signage.

5. Field, A. E., Sonneville, K. R., Crosby, R. D., Swanson, S. A., Eddy, K. T., Camargo, C. A., et al. (2014). Prospective associations of concerns about physique and the development of obesity, binge drinking, and drug use among adolescent boys and young adult men. *JAMA Pediatrics, 168,* 34–39 (p. 37). doi:10.1001/jamapediatrics.2013.2915.

6. Crichton, P. (1996). Were the Roman emperors Claudius and Vitellius bulimic? *International Journal of Eating Disorders, 19,* 203–207 (p. 206).

7. Dr. Tuckwell avoided using the term "hysterical vomiting" because two of his patients were boys and the one girl, although 14, had not yet started menstruating.

8. Access to modern plumbing likely facilitates secretive purging in a way that chamber pots and outhouses would not. An inability to purge privately may have protected many from developing this particular problem for centuries.

9. Salter, H. (1868). Hysterical vomiting. *Lancet, 92,* 164–165; 242–244 (p. 164).

10. These are additional physical symptoms reported in cases of hysterical vomiting that make it seem different from purging disorder.

11. Becker, A. E., Burwell, R. A., Gilman, S. E., Herzog, D. B., & Hamburg, P. (2002). Eating behaviours and attitudes following prolonged exposure to television among ethnic Fijian adolescent girls. *British Journal of Psychiatry, 180,* 509–514 (p. 513).

12. Thomas, J. J., Crosby, R. D., Wonderlich, S. A., Striegel-Moore, R. H., & Becker, A. E. (2011). A latent profile analysis of the typology of bulimic symptoms in an indigenous Pacific population: Evidence of cross-cultural variation in phenomenology. *Psychological Medicine, 41,* 195–206 (p. 198). doi:10.1017/S0033291710000255.

13. Ibid.

14. Morris, P. F., & Szabo, C. P. (2013). Meanings of thinness and dysfunctional eating in black South African females: A qualitative study. *African Journal of Psychiatry, 16,* 338–342. doi:http://dx.doi.org/10.4314/ajpsy.v16i5.45.

CHAPTER 3

1. As noted in chapter 1, the original meaning of purge is to purify.

2. https://www.forbes.com/sites/natalierobehmed/2018/12/13/highest-paid-models-2018-kendall-jenner-leads-with-22-5-million/#2c98646e3ddf

3. Calculations of BMI for individuals listed by *Forbes* magazine were based on statistics drawn from https://healthyceleb.com/. According to the site (https://healthyceleb.com/about-us/), "The content on this website is true to the best of our knowledge and is taken from the celebrity interviews given to periodicals." However, in its disclaimers (https://healthyceleb.com/disclaimer/) this site also acknowledges that "We are not liable / responsible for any wrong, outdated information on HealthyCeleb.com. Though, we try our best to keep the information correct and up to date. Though some of the celeb profiles are written by the celebs themselves, but that would be mentioned in the profile itself. Otherwise, the information provided in the 'Body Statistics' articles is not any personal view of the writer of Healthy Celeb. Those are taken from the celeb's interviews given to various magazines, newspapers, and journals."

4. https://www.cdc.gov/obesity/adult/causes.html

5. To calculate BMI, take body weight in kilograms and then divide that number by the squared value of height in meters. When measuring weight in pounds, and height in inches, BMI = 703 weight [height]^2.

6. Particularly interesting was that the benefits of consuming more fruits and whole grains and less salt far overshadowed the impact of diets with fat, red meat, or sugar-sweetened beverages. GBD 2017 Diet Collaborators. (2019). Health effects of dietary risks in 195 countries, 1990–2017; a systematic analysis for the Global Burden of Disease Study 2017. *Lancet, 393,* 1958–1972.

7. https://www.forbes.com/pictures/5b746648a7ea43757f2c5b56/7-julia-roberts/#3c83648238a4

8. https://www.forbes.com/pictures/5b7b16ada7ea43757f2cb680/8-adam-sandler/#322619df3a57

9. *Avengers Endgame* was released while I was working on this chapter. In this film, Thor is depicted as significantly overweight through the use of a prosthetic beer belly as a form of comedic relief in this otherwise somber film. This follows the use of Thor's bodily perfection in contrast to Starlord's "flabbiness" in *Avengers Infinity Wars* as comedic relief. Both movies directly ridicule weight gain in men while idealizing muscularity.

10. Girls and boys did not differ on how positively they rated the figures overall. Thus, my description focuses on how all children rated figures of girls versus figures of boys.

11. To take the IAT and contribute to ongoing research examining unconscious attitudes across a number of topics, you can visit https://implicit.harvard.edu/implicit/.

12. Charlesworth, T. E. S., & Banaji, M. R. (2019). Patterns of implicit and explicit attitudes: I. Long-term change and stability from 2007 to 2016. *Psychological Science, 30*(2), 174–192.

13. Richardson, S. A., Goodman, N., Hastorf, A. H., & Dornbusch, S. M (1961). Cultural uniformity in reaction to physical disabilities. *American Sociological Review, 26,* 241–247 (p. 243).

14. Interestingly, for boys, importance of weight to peers also predicted who started to purge during seven-year follow-up.

15. Chiodo, J., & Latimer, P. R. (1983). Vomiting as a learned weight-control technique in bulimia. *Journal of Behavior Therapy and Experimental Psychiatry, 14,* 131–135 (pp. 132 and 134).

Chapter 4

1. Johns, N. (2009). *Purging: Rehab diaries.* Seal Press (p. 86).

2. Ibid., p. 167.

3. Ibid., p. 168.

4. Ibid., p. 87.

5. Back then, we used a Palm Pilot. These days, participants download apps to their own smartphones to provide this information to researchers.

6. Up to 1,000 calories consumed prior to purging remain in the body after purging due to the fast absorption of energy throughout the digestive tract.

Chapter 5

1. Brody, J. (2007). Out of control: A true story of binge eating. *New York Times,* February 20.

CHAPTER 6

1. https://nccih.nih.gov/health/detoxes-cleanses
2. Academy for Eating Disorders. (2016). *Eating disorders: A guide to medical care. Critical points for early recognition & medical risk management in the care of individuals with eating disorders* (3rd ed). https://higherlogicdownload. s3.amazonaws.com/AEDWEB/05656ea0-59c9-4dd4-b832-07a3fea58f4c/ UploadedImages/AED_Medical_Care_Guidelines_English_04_03_18_a.pdf

CHAPTER 7

1. For more information on Project Heal go to https://www.eatingdisorderhope.com/ blog/what-resources-are-available-to-help-me-cover-the-cost-of-eating-disorder- treatment.
2. The U.S. Centers for Disease Control and Prevention offers a free online calculator for children and teens in which age, sex, height, and weight can be entered either in inches/pounds or in centimeters/kilograms to provide the age- and sex-adjusted percentile (https://www.cdc.gov/healthyweight/bmi/calculator.html). This online tool also provides a characterization of whether the weight falls inside or outside of a healthy range.
3. This case study was presented in a chapter on purging disorder, co-authored with my students, and represents an amalgamation of patients seen by Dr. K. Jean Forney.
4. DSM-5, pp. 338–339.

CHAPTER 8

1. Sysko, R., & Hildebrandt, T. (2011). Enhanced cognitive behavioral therapy for an adolescent with purging disorder: A case report. *European Eating Disorders Review*, *19*, 37–45 (p. 42).
2. In case you're wondering, outcomes were better for patients with bulimia compared to those with anorexia. This reflect both a greater magnitude of dif- ference (57% vs. 34%) and the larger number of patients. The larger number of patients in each group increases the ability to determine that this difference was statistically significant.
3. Waller, G., Gray, E., Hinrichsen, H., Mountford, V., Lawson, R., & Patient, E. (2014). Cognitive-behavioral therapy for bulimia nervosa and atypical bulimia nervosa: Effectiveness in clinical settings. *International Journal of Eating Disorders*, *47*, 13–17 (p. 15).
4. Fairburn, C. (1981). A cognitive behavioural approach to the treatment of bulimia. *Psychological Medicine, 11*, 707–711 (p. 710).

CHAPTER 9

1. This study isn't included among the follow-up studies described above for two reasons. First, women didn't necessarily have purging disorder at baseline. Instead, diagnosis was based on retrospective report of symptoms. The studies described above all started with women at the time that purging disorder was diagnosed and followed them. Second, all women were pregnant. At any given time, about 3.4% of women are pregnant in the United States, and 0% of men, prepubertal girls, and postmenopausal women are pregnant worldwide. This means that most individuals

with purging disorder aren't pregnant, making findings for pregnant women specific to that group.

2. World Health Organization. International Classification of Diseases 11 for Mortality and Morbidity Statistics 2018. https://icd.who.int/browse11/l-m/en#/http%3a%2f%2fid.who.int%2ficd%2fentity%2f509381842.

SOURCE REFERENCES

Throughout the book, I have drawn from numerous scientific journals articles and books to describe research findings for purging disorder. Below are references for these publications so that you may consult them for additional information not covered in the book.

Academy for Eating Disorders Medical Care Task Force. (2016). *Eating disorders: A guide to medical care. Critical points for early recognition & medical risk management in the care of individuals with eating disorders* (3rd ed.). https://higherlogicdownload. s3.amazonaws.com/AEDWEB/05656ea0-59c9-4dd4-b832-07a3fea58f4c/ UploadedImages/AED_Medical_Care_Guidelines_English_04_03_18_a.pdf

Allen, K. L., Byrne, S. M., Oddy, W. H., & Crosby, R. D. (2013). DSM-IV-TR and DSM-5 eating disorders in adolescents: Prevalence, stability, and psychosocial correlates in a population-based sample of male and female adolescents. *Journal of Abnormal Psychology, 122*(3), 720–732.

American Psychiatric Association. (1980). *Diagnostic and statistical manual of mental disorders* (3rd ed.). American Psychiatric Publishing.

American Psychiatric Association. (1987). *Diagnostic and statistical manual of mental disorders* (3rd ed., rev.). American Psychiatric Publishing.

American Psychiatric Association. (1994). *Diagnostic and statistical manual of mental disorders* (4th ed.). American Psychiatric Publishing.

American Psychiatric Association. (2013). *Diagnostic and statistical manual of mental disorders* (5th ed.). American Psychiatric Publishing.

Austin, S. B., Field, A. E., Wiecha, J., Peterson, K. E., & Gortmaker, S. L. (2005). The impact of a school-based obesity prevention trial on disordered weight-control behaviors in early adolescent girls. *Archives of Pediatrics & Adolescent Medicine, 159*(3), 225–230.

Becker, A. E., Burwell, R. A., Gilman, S. E., Herzog, D. B., & Hamburg, P. (2002). Eating behaviours and attitudes following prolonged exposure to television among ethnic Fijian adolescent girls. *British Journal of Psychiatry, 180*, 509–514.

Becker, A. E., Thomas, J. J., Bainivualiku, A., Richards, L., Navara, K., Roberts, A. L., et al. (2010). Adaptation and evaluation of the clinical impairment assessment to assess disordered eating related distress in an adolescent female ethnic Fijian population. *International Journal of Eating Disorders, 43*(2), 179–186.

Becker, A. E., Thomas, J. J., Bainivualiku, A., Richards, L., Navara, K., Roberts, A. L., et al. (2010). Validity and reliability of a Fijian translation and adaptation of the eating disorder examination questionnaire. *International Journal of Eating Disorders, 43*(2), 171–178.

Becker, C. B., Bull, S., Schaumberg, K., Cauble, A., & Franco, A. (2008). Effectiveness of peer-led eating disorders prevention: A replication trial. *Journal of Consulting and Clinical Psychology, 76*(2), 347–354.

Birgegard, A., Norring, C., & Clinton, D. (2012). DSM-IV versus DSM-5: Implementation of proposed DSM-5 criteria in a large naturalistic database. *International Journal of Eating Disorders, 45*(3), 353–361.

Boron, W. F., & Boulpaep, E. L. (2017). *Medical physiology* (3rd ed.). Elsevier.

Brown, T. A., Forney, K. J., Pinner, D., & Keel, P. K. (2017). A randomized controlled trial of The Body Project: More Than Muscles for men with body dissatisfaction. *International Journal of Eating Disorders, 50*(8), 873–883.

Brown, T. A., Haedt-Matt, A. A., & Keel, P. K. (2011). Personality pathology in purging disorder and bulimia nervosa. *International Journal of Eating Disorders, 44*(8), 735–740.

Bruch, H. (1978). *The golden cage: The enigma of anorexia nervosa.* Harvard University Press.

Bulik, C. M., Blake, L., & Austin, J. (2019). Genetics of eating disorders: What the clinician needs to know. *Psychiatric Clinics of North America, 42*(1), 59–73.

Charlesworth, T. E. S., & Banaji, M. R. (2019). Patterns of implicit and explicit attitudes: I. Long-term change and stability from 2007 to 2016. *Psychological Science, 30*(2), 174–192.

Chiodo, J., & Latimer, P. R. (1983). Vomiting as a learned weight-control technique in bulimia. *Journal of Behavior Therapy and Experimental Psychiatry, 14*(2), 131–135.

Coupland. (1881). Middlesex Hospital: Hysterical vomiting of eight months' duration. *Lancet, 117*(2999), 291–292.

Crichton, P. (1996). Were the Roman emperors Claudius and Vitellius bulimic? *International Journal of Eating Disorders, 19*(2), 203–207.

Crowther, J. H., Armey, M., Luce, K. H., Dalton, G. R., & Leahey, T. (2008). The point prevalence of bulimic disorders from 1990 to 2004. *International Journal of Eating Disorders, 41*(6), 491–497.

Culbert, K. M., Burt, S. A., McGue, M., & Iacono, W. G., & Klump, K. L. (2009). Puberty and the genetic diathesis of disordered eating attitudes and behaviors. *Journal of Abnormal Psychology, 118*(4), 788–796.

Darcy, A. M., Fitzpatrick, K. K., Manasse, S. M., Datta, N., Klabunde, M., Colborn, D., et al. (2015). Central coherence in adolescents with bulimia nervosa spectrum eating disorders. *International Journal of Eating Disorders, 48*(5), 487–493.

Dossat, A. M., Bodell, L. P., Williams, D. L., Eckel, L. A., & Keel, P. K. (2015). Preliminary examination of glucagon-like peptide-1 levels in women with purging disorder and bulimia nervosa. *International Journal of Eating Disorders, 48*(2), 199–205.

Dutton, E. (1888). A severe case of hysteria, cured by massage, seclusion, and over-feeding. *Lancet, 131*(3380), 1128–1129.

Eddy, K. T., Celio Doyle, A., Hoste, R. R., Herzog, D. B., & le Grange, D. (2008). Eating disorder not otherwise specified in adolescents. *Journal of the American Academy of Child and Adolescent Psychiatry, 47*(2), 156–164.

Eddy, K. T., Hennessey, M., & Thompson-Brenner, H. (2007). Eating pathology in East African women: The role of media exposure and globalization. *Journal of Nervous and Mental Disease, 195*(3), 196–202.

Ekeroth, K., Clinton, D., Norring, C., & Birgegard, A. (2013). Clinical characteristics and distinctiveness of DSM-5 eating disorder diagnoses: Findings from a large natural-istic clinical database. *Journal of Eating Disorders, 1*, 31-2974-1-31. eCollection 2013.

Fairburn, C. G. (1980). Self-induced vomiting. *Journal of Psychosomatic Research, 24*(3-4), 193–197.

Fairburn, C. (1981). A cognitive behavioural approach to the treatment of bulimia. *Psychological Medicine, 11*(4), 707–711.

Fairburn, C. (1985). Cognitive-behavioral treatment for bulimia. In Garner, D. M., & Garfinkel, P. E. (eds.), *Handbook of psychotherapy for anorexia nervosa and bulimia* (pp. 160–192). Guilford Press.

Fairburn, C. G., Bailey-Straebler, S., Basden, S., Doll, H. A., Jones, R., Murphy, R., et al. (2015). A transdiagnostic comparison of enhanced cognitive behaviour therapy (CBT-E) and interpersonal psychotherapy in the treatment of eating disorders. *Behaviour Research and Therapy, 70*, 64–71.

Fairburn, C. G., Cooper, Z., Doll, H. A., O'Connor, M. E., Bohn, K., Hawker, D. M., et al. (2009). Transdiagnostic cognitive-behavioral therapy for patients with eating disorders: A two-site trial with 60-week follow-up. *American Journal of Psychiatry, 166*(3), 311–319.

Favaro, A., Ferrara, S., & Santonastaso, P. (2003). The spectrum of eating disorders in young women: A prevalence study in a general population sample. *Psychosomatic Medicine, 65*(4), 701–708.

Field, A. E., Camargo, C. A., Jr, Taylor, C. B., Berkey, C. S., & Colditz, G. A. (1999). Relation of peer and media influences to the development of purging behaviors among preadolescent and adolescent girls. *Archives of Pediatrics & Adolescent Medicine, 153*(11), 1184–1189.

Field, A. E., Javaras, K. M., Aneja, P., Kitos, N., Camargo, C. A., Jr, Taylor, C. B., et al. (2008). Family, peer, and media predictors of becoming eating disordered. *Archives of Pediatrics & Adolescent Medicine, 162*(6), 574–579.

Field, A. E., Sonneville, K. R., Crosby, R. D., Swanson, S. A., Eddy, K. T., Camargo, C. A., Jr, et al. (2014). Prospective associations of concerns about physique and the devel-opment of obesity, binge drinking, and drug use among adolescent boys and young adult men. *JAMA Pediatrics, 168*(1), 34–39.

Field, A. E., Sonneville, K. R., Micali, N., Crosby, R. D., Swanson, S. A., Laird, N. M., et al. (2012). Prospective association of common eating disorders and adverse outcomes. *Pediatrics, 130*(2), e289–e295.

Fink, E. L., Smith, A. R., Gordon, K. H., Holm-Denoma, J. M., & Joiner, T. E. Jr. (2009). Psychological correlates of purging disorder as compared with other eating disorders: An exploratory investigation. *International Journal of Eating Disorders, 42*(1), 31–39.

Forman-Hoffman, V. L., & Cunningham, C. L. (2008). Geographical clustering of eating disordered behaviors in U.S. high school students. *International Journal of Eating Disorders, 41*(3), 209–214.

Forney, K. J., Buchman-Schmitt, J. M., Keel, P. K., & Frank, G. K. (2016). The medical complications associated with purging. *International Journal of Eating Disorders, 49*(3), 249–259.

Forney, K. J., Crosby, R. D., Brown, T. A., Klein, K. M., & Keel, P. K. (2020). A natural-istic, long-term follow-up of purging disorder. *Psychological Medicine*, Jan. 15.

Forney, K. J., Haedt-Matt, A. A., & Keel, P. K. (2014). The role of loss of control eating in purging disorder. *International Journal of Eating Disorders, 47*(3), 244–251.

Frisch, M. J., Herzog, D. B., & Franko, D. L. (2006). Residential treatment for eating disorders. *International Journal of Eating Disorders, 39*(5), 434–442.

GBD 2017 Diet Collaborators. (2019). Health effects of dietary risks in 195 countries, 1990–2017: A systematic analysis for the global burden of disease study 2017. *Lancet, 393*(10184), 1958–1972.

Giebisch, G., Windhager, E. E., & Aronson, P. S. (2017). Integration of salt and water balance. In W. F. Boron & E. L. Boulpaep (Eds.), *Medical physiology* (3rd ed., pp. 836–849). Elsevier.

Glazer, K. B., Sonneville, K. R., Micali, N., Swanson, S. A., Crosby, R., Horton, N. J., et al. (2019). The course of eating disorders involving bingeing and purging among adolescent girls: Prevalence, stability, and transitions. *Journal of Adolescent Health, 64*(2), 165–171.

Grover, V. P., Keel, P. K., & Mitchell, J. P. (2003). Gender differences in implicit weight identity. *International Journal of Eating Disorders, 34*(1), 125–135.

Haedt, A. A., & Keel, P. K. (2010). Comparing definitions of purging disorder on point prevalence and associations with external validators. *International Journal of Eating Disorders, 43*(5), 433–439.

Haedt-Matt, A. A., & Keel, P. K. (2015). Affect regulation and purging: An ecological momentary assessment study in purging disorder. *Journal of Abnormal Psychology, 124*(2), 399–411.

Hammerle, F., Huss, M., Ernst, V., & Burger, A. (2016). Thinking dimensional: Prevalence of DSM-5 early adolescent full syndrome, partial and subthreshold eating disorders in a cross-sectional survey in German schools. *BMJ Open, 6*(5), e010843-2015-010843.

Hay, P. J., Mond, J., Buttner, P., & Darby, A. (2008). Eating disorder behaviors are increasing: Findings from two sequential community surveys in South Australia. *PloS One, 3*(2), e1541.

Himmerich, H., Bentley, J., Kan, C., & Treasure, J. (2019). Genetic risk factors for eating disorders: An update and insights into pathophysiology. *Therapeutic Advances in Psychopharmacology, 9*, 2045125318814734.

Johns, N. (2009). *Purge: Rehab diaries.* Hachette UK.

Kaye, W. H., Weltzin, T. E., Hsu, L. K., McConaha, C. W., & Bolton, B. (1993). Amount of calories retained after binge eating and vomiting. *American Journal of Psychiatry, 150*(6), 969–971.

Kazmi, N., Gaunt, T. R., Relton, C., & Micali, N. (2017). Maternal eating disorders affect offspring cord blood DNA methylation: A prospective study. *Clinical Epigenetics, 9*, 120-017-0418-3. eCollection 2017.

Keel, P. K. (2007). Purging disorder: Subthreshold variant or full-threshold eating disorder? *International Journal of Eating Disorders, 40*(S3), S89–S94.

Keel, P. K. (2017). *Eating disorders* (2nd ed.). Oxford University Press.

Keel, P. K. (2019). Purging disorder: Recent advances and future challenges. *Current Opinion in Psychiatry, 32*(6), 518–524.

Keel, P. K., Eckel, L. A., Hildebrandt, B. A., Haedt-Matt, A. A., Appelbaum, J., & Jimerson, D. C. (2018). Disturbance of gut satiety peptide in purging disorder. *International Journal of Eating Disorders, 51*(1), 53–61.

Keel, P. K., Haedt, A., & Edler, C. (2005). Purging disorder: An ominous variant of bulimia nervosa? *International Journal of Eating Disorders*, 38(3), 191–199.

Keel, P. K., Haedt-Matt, A. A., Hildebrandt, B., Bodell, L. P., Wolfe, B. E., & Jimerson, D. C. (2018). Satiation deficits and binge eating: Probing differences between bulimia nervosa and purging disorder using an ad lib test meal. *Appetite*, 127, 119–125.

Keel, P. K., Holm-Denoma, J. M., & Crosby, R. D. (2011). Clinical significance and distinctiveness of purging disorder and binge eating disorder. *International Journal of Eating Disorders*, 44(4), 311–316.

Keel, P. K., & Klump, K. L. (2003). Are eating disorders culture-bound syndromes? implications for conceptualizing their etiology. *Psychological Bulletin*, 129(5), 747.

Keel, P. K., Mayer, S. A., & Harnden-Fischer, J. H. (2001). Importance of size in defining binge eating episodes in bulimia nervosa. *International Journal of Eating Disorders*, 29(3), 294–301.

Keel, P. K., & Mitchell, J. E. (1997). Outcome in bulimia nervosa. *American Journal of Psychiatry*, 154(3), 313–321.

Keel, P. K., Mitchell, J. E., Miller, K. B., Davis, T. L., & Crow, S. J. (1999). Long-term outcome of bulimia nervosa. *Archives of General Psychiatry*, 56(1), 63–69.

Keel, P. K., & Striegel-Moore, R. H. (2009). The validity and clinical utility of purging disorder. *International Journal of Eating Disorders*, 42(8), 706–719.

Keel, P. K., Wolfe, B. E., Gravener, J. A., & Jimerson, D. C. (2008). Co-morbidity and disorder-related distress and impairment in purging disorder. *Psychological Medicine*, 38(10), 1435–1442.

Keel, P. K., Wolfe, B. E., Liddle, R. A., De Young, K. P., & Jimerson, D. C. (2007). Clinical features and physiological response to a test meal in purging disorder and bulimia nervosa. *Archives of General Psychiatry*, 64(9), 1058–1066.

Kennedy, G. A., Klein, K. M., & Keel, P. K. (2018). Prevalence and predictors of parental concern for children's weight from 2002 to 2012. *Public Health*, 162, 58–62.

Klein, K. M., Brown, T. A., Kennedy, G. A., & Keel, P. K. (2017). Examination of parental dieting and comments as risk factors for increased drive for thinness in men and women at 20-year follow-up. *International Journal of Eating Disorders*, 50(5), 490–497.

Klump, K. L., Culbert, K. M., Slane, J. D., Burt, S. A., Sisk, C. L., & Nigg, J. T. (2012). The effects of puberty on genetic risk for disordered eating: evidence for a sex difference. *Psychological Medicine*, 42(3), 627–637.

Klump, K. L., McGue, M., & Iacono, W. G. (2000). Age differences in genetic and environmental influences on eating attitudes and behaviors in preadolescent and adolescent female twins. *Journal of Abnormal Psychology*, 109(2), 239–251.

Klump, K. L., McGue, M., & Iacono, W. G. (2002). Genetic relationships between personality and eating attitudes and behaviors. *Journal of Abnormal Psychology*, 111(2), 380–389.

Knoph, C., Von Holle, A., Zerwas, S., Torgersen, L., Tambs, K., Stoltenberg, C., et al. (2013). Course and predictors of maternal eating disorders in the postpartum period. *International Journal of Eating Disorders*, 46(4), 355–368.

Koch, S., Quadflieg, N., & Fichter, M. (2013). Purging disorder: A comparison to established eating disorders with purging behaviour. *European Eating Disorders Review*, 21(4), 265–275.

Koch, S., Quadflieg, N., & Fichter, M. (2014). Purging disorder: A pathway to death? A review of 11 cases. *Eating and Weight Disorders, 19*(1), 21–29.

Kraig, K. A., & Keel, P. K. (2001). Weight-based stigmatization in children. *International Journal of Obesity, 25*(11), 1661.

Lavender, J. M., Utzinger, L. M., Cao, L., Wonderlich, S. A., Engel, S. G., Mitchell, J. E., et al. (2016). Reciprocal associations between negative affect, binge eating, and purging in the natural environment in women with bulimia nervosa. *Journal of Abnormal Psychology, 125*(3), 381–386.

le Grange, D., Crosby, R. D., Rathouz, P. J., & Leventhal, B. L. (2007). A randomized controlled comparison of family-based treatment and supportive psychotherapy for adolescent bulimia nervosa. *Archives of General Psychiatry, 64*(9), 1049–1056.

Lowe, M. R., Piers, A. D., & Benson, L. (2018). Weight suppression in eating disorders: A research and conceptual update. *Current Psychiatry Reports, 20*(10), 80–018-0955-2.

Mabe, A. G., Forney, K. J., & Keel, P. K. (2014). Do you "like" my photo? Facebook use maintains eating disorder risk. *International Journal of Eating Disorders, 47*(5), 516–523.

MacDonald, D. E., McFarlane, T. L., Dionne, M. M., David, L., & Olmsted, M. P. (2017). Rapid response to intensive treatment for bulimia nervosa and purging disorder: A randomized controlled trial of a CBT intervention to facilitate early behavior change. *Journal of Consulting and Clinical Psychology, 85*(9), 896–908.

Mantel, A., Hirschberg, A. L., & Stephansson, O. (2019). Association of maternal eating disorders with pregnancy and neonatal outcomes. *JAMA Psychiatry*, Nov. 20.

McCarthy, L. P., & Gerring, J. P. (1994). Revising psychiatry's charter document: DSM-IV. *Written Communication, 11*(2), 147–192.

Micali, N., Crous-Bou, M., Treasure, J., & Lawson, E. A. (2017). Association between oxytocin receptor genotype, maternal care, and eating disorder behaviours in a community sample of women. *European Eating Disorders Review, 25*(1), 19–25.

Micali, N., Solmi, F., Horton, N. J., Crosby, R. D., Eddy, K. T., Calzo, J. P., et al. (2015). Adolescent eating disorders predict psychiatric, high-risk behaviors and weight outcomes in young adulthood. *Journal of the American Academy of Child and Adolescent Psychiatry, 54*(8), 652–659.

Mitchell, J. E., Pyle, R. L., Hatsukami, D., & Eckert, E. D. (1986). What are atypical eating disorders? *Psychosomatics, 27*(1), 21–28.

Mitchison, D., Mond, J., Bussey, K., Griffiths, S., Trompeter, N., Lonergan, A., et al. (2019). DSM-5 full syndrome, other specified, and unspecified eating disorders in Australian adolescents: Prevalence and clinical significance. *Psychological Medicine*, May 2.

Morris, P., & Szabo, C. (2013). Meanings of thinness and dysfunctional eating in black South African females: A qualitative study. *African Journal of Psychiatry, 16*(5), 338–342.

Munn-Chernoff, M. A., Keel, P. K., Klump, K. L., Grant, J. D., Bucholz, K. K., Madden, P. A., et al. (2015). Prevalence of and familial influences on purging disorder in a community sample of female twins. *International Journal of Eating Disorders, 48*(6), 601–606.

Nakai, Y., Nin, K., Noma, S., Teramukai, S., Fujikawa, K., & Wonderlich, S. A. (2018). Changing profile of eating disorders between 1963 and 2004 in a Japanese sample. *International Journal of Eating Disorders, 51*(8), 953–958.

Peebles, R., Lesser, A., Park, C. C., Heckert, K., Timko, C. A., Lantzouni, E., et al. (2017). Outcomes of an inpatient medical nutritional rehabilitation protocol in children and adolescents with eating disorders. *Journal of Eating Disorders*, 5, 7-017-0134-6. eCollection 2017.

Peterson, C. B., Miller, K. B., Willer, M. G., Ziesmer, J., Durkin, N., Arikian, A., et al. (2011). Cognitive-behavioral therapy for subthreshold bulimia nervosa: A case series. *Eating and Weight Disorders*, 16(3), e204–208.

Peterson, C. M., Baker, J. H., Thornton, L. M., Trace, S. E., Mazzeo, S. E., Neale, M. C., et al. (2016). Genetic and environmental components to self-induced vomiting. *International Journal of Eating Disorders*, 49(4), 421–427.

Pisetsky, E. M., Thornton, L. M., Lichtenstein, P., Pedersen, N. L., & Bulik, C. M. (2013). Suicide attempts in women with eating disorders. *Journal of Abnormal Psychology*, 122(4), 1042–1056.

Richardson, S. A., Goodman, N., Hastorf, A. H., & Dornbusch, S. M. (1961). Cultural uniformity in reaction to physical disabilities. *American Sociological Review*, 26, 241–247.

Riesco, N., Aguera, Z., Granero, R., Jimenez-Murcia, S., Menchon, J. M., & Fernandez-Aranda, F. (2018). Other specified feeding or eating disorders (OSFED): Clinical heterogeneity and cognitive-behavioral therapy outcome. *European Psychiatry*, 54, 109–116.

Roberto, C. A., Grilo, C. M., Masheb, R. M., & White, M. A. (2010). Binge eating, purging, or both: Eating disorder psychopathology findings from an internet community survey. *International Journal of Eating Disorders*, 43(8), 724–731.

Russell, G. (1979). Bulimia nervosa: An ominous variant of anorexia nervosa. *Psychological Medicine*, 9(3), 429–448.

Salter, H. (1868). Clinical lecture on hysterical vomiting. *Lancet*, 92(2340), 1–2, 37–38.

Sancho, C., Arija, M., Asorey, O., & Canals, J. (2007). Epidemiology of eating disorders. *European Child & Adolescent Psychiatry*, 16(8), 495–504.

Schmidt, U., Lee, S., Beecham, J., Perkins, S., Treasure, J., Yi, I., et al. (2007). A randomized controlled trial of family therapy and cognitive behavior therapy guided self-care for adolescents with bulimia nervosa and related disorders. *American Journal of Psychiatry*, 164(4), 591–598.

Silventoinen, K., Jelenkovic, A., Sund, R., Hur, Y. M., Yokoyama, Y., Honda, C., et al. (2016). Genetic and environmental effects on body mass index from infancy to the onset of adulthood: An individual-based pooled analysis of 45 twin cohorts participating in the Collaborative Project of Development of Anthropometrical Measures in Twins (CODATwins) study. *American Journal of Clinical Nutrition*, 104(2), 371–379.

Smith, K. E., & Crowther, J. H. (2013). An exploratory investigation of purging disorder. *Eating Behaviors*, 14(1), 26–34.

Solmi, F., Hotopf, M., Hatch, S., Treasure, J., & Micali, N. (2016). Eating disorders in a multi-ethnic inner-city UK sample: Prevalence, comorbidity and service use. *Social Psychiatry and Psychiatric Epidemiology*, 51(3), 369–381.

Stice, E., & Desjardins, C. D. (2018). Interactions between risk factors in the prediction of onset of eating disorders: Exploratory hypothesis generating analyses. *Behaviour Research and Therapy*, 105, 52–62.

Stice, E., Gau, J. M., Rohde, P., & Shaw, H. (2017). Risk factors that predict future onset of each DSM-5 eating disorder: Predictive specificity in high-risk adolescent females. *Journal of Abnormal Psychology, 126*(1), 38–51.

Stice, E., Marti, C. N., & Rohde, P. (2013). Prevalence, incidence, impairment, and course of the proposed DSM-5 eating disorder diagnoses in an 8-year prospective community study of young women. *Journal of Abnormal Psychology, 122*(2), 445.

Striegel-Moore, R. H., Leslie, D., Petrill, S. A., Garvin, V., & Rosenheck, R. A. (2000). One-year use and cost of inpatient and outpatient services among female and male patients with an eating disorder: Evidence from a national database of health insurance claims. *International Journal of Eating Disorders, 27*(4), 381–389.

Swanson, S. A., Brown, T. A., Crosby, R. D., & Keel, P. K. (2014). What are we missing? The costs versus benefits of skip rule designs. *International Journal of Methods in Psychiatric Research, 23*(4), 474–485.

Sysko, R., & Hildebrandt, T. (2011). Enhanced cognitive behavioural therapy for an adolescent with purging disorder: A case report. *European Eating Disorders Review, 19*(1), 37–45.

Tasca, G. A., Maxwell, H., Bone, M., Trinneer, A., Balfour, L., & Bissada, H. (2012). Purging disorder: Psychopathology and treatment outcomes. *International Journal of Eating Disorders, 45*(1), 36–42.

Thomas, J. J., Crosby, R. D., Wonderlich, S. A., Striegel-Moore, R. H., & Becker, A. E. (2011). A latent profile analysis of the typology of bulimic symptoms in an indigenous pacific population: Evidence of cross-cultural variation in phenomenology. *Psychological Medicine, 41*(1), 195–206.

Thornton, L. M., Mazzeo, S. E., & Bulik, C. M. (2011). The heritability of eating disorders: Methods and current findings. *Current Topics in Behavioral Neurosciences, 6*, 141–156.

Torgersen, L., Von Holle, A., Reichborn-Kjennerud, T., Berg, C. K., Hamer, R., Sullivan, P., et al. (2008). Nausea and vomiting of pregnancy in women with bulimia nervosa and eating disorders not otherwise specified. *International Journal of Eating Disorders, 41*(8), 722–727.

Tuckwell, H. M. (1873). On vomiting of habit. *British Medical Journal, 1*(638), 310–311.

Vo, M., Accurso, E. C., Goldschmidt, A. B., & Le Grange, D. (2017). The impact of DSM-5 on eating disorder diagnoses. *International Journal of Eating Disorders, 50*(5), 578–581.

Wade, T. D., Bergin, J. L., Tiggemann, M., Bulik, C. M., & Fairburn, C. G. (2006). Prevalence and long-term course of lifetime eating disorders in an adult Australian twin cohort. *Australian and New Zealand Journal of Psychiatry, 40*(2), 121–128.

Wade, T. D., Treloar, S., & Martin, N. G. (2008). Shared and unique risk factors between lifetime purging and objective binge eating: A twin study. *Psychological Medicine, 38*(10), 1455–1464.

Waller, G. (2016). Treatment protocols for eating disorders: Clinicians' attitudes, concerns, adherence and difficulties delivering evidence-based psychological interventions. *Current Psychiatry Reports, 18*(4), 36-016-0679-0.

Waller, G., Gray, E., Hinrichsen, H., Mountford, V., Lawson, R., & Patient, E. (2014). Cognitive-behavioral therapy for bulimia nervosa and atypical bulimic nervosa: Effectiveness in clinical settings. *International Journal of Eating Disorders, 47*(1), 13–17.

Watson, H. J., Diemer, E. W., Zerwas, S., Gustavson, K., Knudsen, G. P., Torgersen, L., et al. (2019). Prenatal and perinatal risk factors for eating disorders in women: A population cohort study. *International Journal of Eating Disorders, 52*(6), 643–651.

Watson, H. J., Torgersen, L., Zerwas, S., Reichborn-Kjennerud, T., Knoph, C., Stoltenberg, C., et al. (2014). Eating disorders, pregnancy, and the postpartum period: Findings from the Norwegian mother and child cohort study (MoBa). *Norwegian Journal of Epidemiology, 24*(1-2), 51–62.

Watson, H. J., Yilmaz, Z., Thornton, L. M., Hubel, C., Coleman, J. R. I., Gaspar, H. A., et al. (2019). Genome-wide association study identifies eight risk loci and implicates metabo-psychiatric origins for anorexia nervosa. *Nature Genetics, 51*(8), 1207–1214.

Wick, M. R., & Keel, P. K. (in press). Posting edited photos of the self: increasing eating disorder risk or harmless behavior? *International Journal of Eating Disorders.*

Wonderlich, S. A., Peterson, C. B., Crosby, R. D., Smith, T. L., Klein, M. H., Mitchell, J. E., et al. (2014). A randomized controlled comparison of integrative cognitive-affective therapy (ICAT) and enhanced cognitive-behavioral therapy (CBT-E) for bulimia nervosa. *Psychological Medicine, 44*(3), 543–553.

Yilmaz, Z., Gottfredson, N. C., Zerwas, S. C., Bulik, C. M., & Micali, N. (2019). Developmental premorbid body mass index trajectories of adolescents with eating disorders in a longitudinal population cohort. *Journal of the American Academy of Child and Adolescent Psychiatry, 58*(2), 191–199.

ADDITIONAL RESOURCES

The following alphabetical list of resources presents recommendations from those who study, treat, or have been affected by eating disorders. The summary does not represent an endorsement of listed resources and does not represent a complete or comprehensive list of all available or useful resources.

FOR THOSE WHO PURGE

Books

Bulik, C. M. (2013). *Midlife eating disorders: Your journey to recovery* Bloomsbury Publishing USA.

Cash, T. (2008). *The body image workbook: An eight-step program for learning to like your looks.* New Harbinger Publications.

Costin, C., & Grabb, G. S. (2011). *8 keys to recovery from an eating disorder: Effective strategies from therapeutic practice and personal experience (8 keys to mental health).* WW Norton & Company.

Thomas, J. J., & Schaefer, J. (2013). *Almost anorexic: Is my (or my loved one's) relationship with food a problem?* Hazelden Publishing.

Online Resources

- Tabitha Farrar's Eating Disorder Recovery for Adults: https://tabithafarrar.com/
- Project Heal website for online communities and grants for treatment access: https://www.theprojectheal.org/
- UCSD's Recipes for Recovery: https://ucsdeatingdisorders.tumblr.com/post/70598642176/recipes-for-recovery
- A message of hope via A2AStories: http://a2aalliance.org/a2a-spotlight/a2a-spotlight-kelsey-heenan/
- One-minute medical videos for patients: https://www.youtube.com/channel/UCf_ucSN36uUJRY06f7sbydA
- Bhuddify Meditation and Mindfulness app: https://buddhify.com/

For Parents, Family, Friends, and Supporters

Books

Lock, J., & Le Grange, D. (2015). *Help your teenager beat an eating disorder.* Guilford Publications.

Muhlheim, L. (2018). *When your teen has an eating disorder: Practical strategies to help your teen recover from anorexia, bulimia, and binge eating.* New Harbinger Publications.

Neumark-Sztainer, D. (2005). *I'm, like, SO fat!: Helping your teen make healthy choices about eating and exercise in a weight-obsessed world.* Guilford Press.

Treasure, J., Smith, G., & Crane, A. (2016). *Skills-based caring for a loved one with an eating disorder: The new Maudsley method.* Routledge.

Online Resources

- National Eating Disorders Association parent tookit: https://www.nationaleatingdisorders.org/parent-toolkit
- Support for siblings of those with eating disorders: https://www.kymadvocates.com/
- FEAST Around the Dinner Table Forum (a moderated online discussion for parents, families, and supporters of patients with eating disorders): https://www.feast-ed.org/around-the-dinner-table-forum/
- Parents using the Maudsley family treatment method: http://www.maudsleyparents.org/

For General Practitioners (Not Eating Disorder Specialists)

Books

Anderson, L. K., Murray, S. B., & Kaye, W. H. (2017). *Clinical handbook of complex and atypical eating disorders.* Oxford University Press.

Lock, J. (2018). *Pocket guide for the assessment and treatment of eating disorders.* American Psychiatric Publishing.

Online Resources

- "The science behind the Academy for Eating Disorders' *Nine truths about eating disorders*" (2017) by Katherine Schaumberg and colleagues: https://www.ncbi.nlm.nih.gov/pmc/articles/PMC5711426/
- Center for Clinical Interventions: https://www.cci.health.wa.gov.au/Resources/For-Clinicians/Eating-Disorders
- "Eating disorders: Recognition and treatment" from the National Institute for Health and Care Excellence: https://www.nice.org.uk/guidance/ng69
- Academy for Eating Disorders, *Eating disorders: A guide to medical care*: https://www.aedweb.org/resources/publications/medical-care-standards

For Eating Disorder Professionals

Books

Deliberto, T. L., & Hirsch, D. (2019). *Treating eating disorders in adolescents: Evidence-based interventions for anorexia, bulimia, and binge eating.* New Harbinger Publications.

Linehan, M. (2014). *DBT skills training manual.* Guilford Publications.

Linehan, M. (2014). *DBT skills training handouts and worksheets.* Guilford Publications.

Lock, J., & Le Grange, D. (2015). *Treatment manual for anorexia nervosa: A family-based approach.* Guilford Publications.

Lynch, T. R. (2018). *Radically open dialectical behavior therapy: Theory and practice for treating disorders of overcontrol.* New Harbinger Publications.

Waller, G., Turner, H., Tatham, M., Mountford, V. A., & Wade, T. D. (2019). *Brief cognitive behavioural therapy for non-underweight patients: CBT-T for eating disorders.* Routledge.

Wonderlich, S. A., Peterson, C. B., & Smith, T. L. (2015). *Integrative cognitive-affective therapy for bulimia nervosa: A treatment manual.* Guilford Publications.

Online Resources

- American Psychological Association, Division 12, Society of Clinical Psychology, Psychological Diagnoses and Other Targets of Treatment, with links for anorexia nervosa, bulimia nervosa, binge-eating disorder, and eating disorders (each link provides evidence base for treatment and links to treatment manuals and training opportunities): https://www.div12.org/diagnoses/
- Workshop presentations for eating disorder treatment: https://www.katetchanturia.com/clinical-work-packages--protocols
- Treatment manuals and publications for eating disorder treatment, with focus on cognitive remediation therapy for anorexia nervosa: https://www.katetchanturia.com/publications
- Centre for Research on Eating Disorders at Oxford (Credo-Oxford) provides information on enhanced cognitive-behavioral therapy (CBT-E), including free access to online training program for CBT-E, guidebooks, handouts, measures, and networking opportunities: https://www.cbte.co/

Training Workshops

- Webinar series on various topics from the Academy for Eating Disorders (reduced fees for members, and some content only available with membership): https://www.aedweb.org/resources/webinars
- Acceptance commitment therapy training from Duke University: https://www.actatduke.org/

For Advanced Specialists

Forsberg, S., Lock, J., & Le Grange, D. (2018). *Family-based treatment for restrictive eating disorders: A guide for supervision and advanced clinical practice.* Routledge.

For Anyone

Any of the above resources may be useful outside their listed group.

Books

Gaudiani, J. L. (2018). *Sick enough: A guide to the medical complications of eating disorders.* Routledge.

Online Resources

- Beat Eating Disorders website: https://www.beateatingdisorders.org.uk/
- Freed from Eating Disorders website: https://freedfromed.co.uk/
- King's College Eating Disorders Research website: https://www.kcl.ac.uk/ioppn/depts/pm/research/eatingdisorders/index
- National Eating Disorders Association website: https://www.nationaleatingdisorders.org/
- Academy for Eating Disorders website: https://www.aedweb.org/home
- Food Psych podcast hosted by Christy Harrison, available through iTunes, Spotify, and https://tunein.com/podcasts/Food/Food-Psych-p553540/
- Eva Musby's YouTube channel: https://www.youtube.com/evamusby
- YoungMinds website for resources to support mental health in children and adolescents, including online articles and blog posts on eating disorders and information on training courses: https://youngminds.org.uk/
- YoungMinds YouTube channel for videos on mental health for children and adolescents: https://www.youtube.com/channel/UCBrcD2CYLBN8v9c7fxRqQAw

Pamela K. Keel, Ph.D., is Distinguished Research Professor and Director of the Eating Behaviors Research Clinic in the Department of Psychology at Florida State University. She received her A.B. in Anthropology *summa cum laude* from Harvard University in 1992 and her Ph.D. in Clinical Psychology from the University of Minnesota in 1998 and completed her clinical psychology internship at Duke University Medical Center in 1998. Dr. Keel has received grants from the National Institutes of Health (NIH) for her research on eating disorders and is co-Principal Investigator and co-Director of the NIMH-funded Integrated Clinical Neuroscience Training Program at Florida State University. She has authored over 200 papers and several books on eating disorders. Dr. Keel defined and characterized purging disorder as a potentially new disorder of eating, and this work contributed to the inclusion of purging disorder as an Other Specified Feeding or Eating Disorder in the *Diagnostic and Statistical Manual of Mental Disorders*, fifth edition (DSM-5). Dr. Keel is a Fellow of the Academy for Eating Disorders (AED), the Association for Psychological Science (APS), and the American Psychological Association (APA). She served as President for the Eating Disorders Research Society and President for the Academy for Eating Disorders. In 2019, Dr. Keel received the Leadership Award in Research from the Academy for Eating Disorders in recognition of an internationally respected body of research yielding new knowledge about eating disorders and measurably advancing the field.

Figures and boxes are indicated by *f* and *b* following the page number

For the benefit of digital users, indexed terms that span two pages (e.g., 52–53) may, on occasion, appear on only one of those pages.